JAILHOUSE DOC

A Doctor in the County Jail

WILLIAM WRIGHT, M.D.

www.williamwrightbooks.com

The people and events in this book are real. Since the characters sometimes lack a sense of humor, I've changed many of the names.

ISBN: 978-1-62967-031-7

Interior formatting by Veronica Yager.
Cover design by Amy Liu.

To Mollie, the keeper of dreams.

CONTENTS

INTRODUCTION

Andy Griffith doesn't work at the El Paso County Jail. Visions of Mayberry quickly vanished amid a flood of addicts, homeless derelicts, and criminals of all stripes. *What the hell was I doing here?*

I used to be an ear surgeon, but after three decades of private practice, I was burned out. I wanted something different, something where I could make a difference. Nine years ago I saw an ad from the Colorado Department of Corrections looking for a physician for the state's maximum-security prison in Cañon City. Well, *that* was different.

My first book, Maximum Insecurity, detailed my life in the supermax, treating the state's most violent and predatory criminals. One day I got a call: "Would you like to be Medical Director at the county jail?" Fateful words that changed the course of my medical career.

I was happy enough in my job caring for inmates in Colorado prisons, but working at the jail would eliminate a long commute, and it paid better. I figured that after the supermax, taking care of a county jail would be a piece of cake.

I thought jails and prisons were pretty much the same, but I quickly discovered that I needed a whole new set of skills. I never knew what was going to walk or be carried into the clinic. It was like running a third-world emergency room.

Some things were familiar from my prison work. I couldn't trust anything my patients told me. I watched constantly for situations that could lead to violence. I learned the ins and outs of the newest and oldest scams.

I faced new challenges caring for patients withdrawing from multiple substances, seeing acutely and chronically ill street people who'd never been to a doctor, and working in a politically charged atmosphere of intimidation and corruption. Not quite what the brochure advertised.

I found an environment of desperate people fresh from the streets ruled by a corrupt sheriff and his concubine sidekick who wanted to take over the medical clinic. If you can't wait to read the juicy details, skip to chapter twenty-six right away.

Jailhouse Doc

We're fascinated by jails, prisons, and medicine. All are institutions that most of us, thankfully, never get to experience from the inside. Here's your chance.

ONE

WHAT'S A NICE BOY LIKE YOU DOING IN A PLACE LIKE THIS?

When anyone gets arrested in El Paso County they quickly end up at the Criminal Justice Center in Colorado Springs, otherwise known as the county jail. I was the Medical Director of CJC, which means I supervised medical care for its 1,500 residents. Being the only physician, the supervision was that much easier.

A career in correctional medicine wasn't tops on my list when I graduated from medical school. I started out as a neuro-otologist, a "super specialist" somewhere between an ear doctor and a neurosurgeon.

This was great for over three decades, but gradually I'd seen everything, done everything, got the T-shirt, and saw the movie as far as treating ear disease was concerned. I was burned out. I did the only sensible thing and retired. Bad mistake.

My wife, Mollie, delicate and lovely creature that she is, fully supported my decision—for the first month. Then I started to get in her hair. Bored, underfoot, I started looking for something different to do. The Colorado Department of Corrections was advertising for a doctor to be the medico at the Colorado State Penitentiary (CSP), the state's maximum security prison. That sounded interesting and kind of exotic with a whiff of Sam Spade danger. It intrigued me.

Mollie pointed out that I knew nothing about being a prison doctor, but I could sense her protestations were feeble. I would be doing something constructive again…elsewhere. I signed up. It turned out that I was pretty good at this stuff.

I was minding my own business at the prison when I was offered the Medical Director position at CJC under mysterious circumstances. Wendy, the Health Services Administrator (HSA) at CJC, gave me a call. Would I be interested? Well, sure. Better pay, no long commute to Cañon City where the prisons were located. Why not? I said I'd like to take a look at the clinic.

Well, that would be great, she said, but could I meet her and Denise, the Director of Nursing (DON), over in the coroner's office instead? Meeting at the clinic just wasn't good right now. Hmm, sure.

I'd envisioned rubbing elbows with the recently deceased during the meeting, but it turned out to be just a plain vanilla classroom without a whiff of formaldehyde. Wendy, a short high-energy blonde, grilled me about my qualifications and experience, while Denise, a taller brunette, played good cop.

After I'd passed enough hurdles to actually be considered a candidate for the job, the pair told me that the reason we couldn't go to the clinic right now was that the doctor I was to replace hadn't actually been fired yet, and they wanted to avoid "unpleasantness."

I was all for that, especially if my soon-to-be-predecessor was bigger than me. We made another appointment to tour the clinic at a neutral time, and I started through the corporate paperwork to get hired. I either gave a hell of an interview, or they were desperate. I'd like to think it was my winning personality and incredible good looks that sealed the deal. I'd like to think that...

Well down the road to getting the new position, I began, belatedly, to think about the job itself. I'd worked at all security levels of prisons for years; how hard could it be to take on a county jail? Little did I know.

When I thought of a county jail, I had visions of Andy Griffith and Mayberry. I looked forward to a low-stress environment where I could sit back and chat with the boys. Maybe go fishin' in the afternoon.

CJC is a little different from that picture. Originally built in the 1980s to house 384 prisoners, the capacity was doubled in 1984 to house 735. Crime being popular in the Springs, occupancy increased by about a hundred each year, so in 1994 a question was put on the ballot to raise funds for a bigger jail.

Colorado Springs residents, conservative to a fault, went to the polls and said "No." In fact they said "Hell, no," by a 3 to 1 majority. By 2002 the occupancy had risen to 1,106 in a facility designed for 735. Things were getting tense.

In 2003 the voters grudgingly sprung for a $32 million expansion consisting of a three-story circular tower that upped capacity to 1,500 beds. It's an odd-looking facility reminiscent of a nuclear plant cooling tower or a sports stadium with a crummy view. The tiny windows sprinkled around the periphery of the cylindrical building remind me of an old player piano roll, albeit a really big one made of cement.

The reason for the circular design is for line-of-sight inside the housing tiers. A deputy in a central control center can directly see each of the four dayrooms in his area. There aren't any corners in which to hide.

When I got my orientation tour of the place, the lack of rectangular structure was a little disorienting, kind of like being inside a huge gerbil wheel. Each housing unit was like a section of an orange, with the control area facing an open common room lined on the outside with two tiers of cells. Between each pair of housing units a recreation area with a basketball court took up part of the perimeter.

Unlike inmates in the state's prisons, the people incarcerated at CJC weren't really inmates or convicts. Most were arrested but hadn't been to court, so they weren't convicted of anything yet. The whole "presumed innocent" thing kicks in, severely restricting what you can and can't do to the detainees. In prison I treated inmates. At CJC I treated patients, just like on the outside in private practice. Pretty much.

An example might help. If Joe is in prison and decides that sticking foreign objects up his nether regions is a fun pastime, we can slap Joe into four-point spread-eagle butt-naked restraints faster than you can say civil rights. But if Joe is in the jail waiting for his court date and he pulls the same stunt, about the best we can do is take away everything we think he might use for that purpose and stick him in a cell by himself. Believe me, it doesn't work nearly as well.

The jail environment differs from prison in many ways, but especially in the amount of drama. In prison, things are settled. Inmates are convicted, sentenced, and assigned to a permanent facility. All the yelling and screaming and protestations of innocence have subsided. Nobody's going anywhere.

At the jail it wasn't so tranquil. Fresh from a crime scene or sleeping under a bridge, persons of all station flowed into CJC. Scared, disoriented, strung-out, drunk, pissed off, sick, beat up arrivals were the norm. These were my patients.

Seeing an incarcerated patient differs quite a bit from dealing with my former private practice patients. With most prisoners there's a layer of anger, fear, and hostility to get past before I could even begin to address their problems. They didn't want to be in this situation, and I was part of the situation they didn't want to be in.

In jail there was the added impediment of an acute change for the worse in their social situation. People in prison have had a chance to adjust, but new jail arrivals are dealing with the shock of being thrown into the slammer, cut off from family and friends.

Add to this social disorientation the very real medical problems they've dragged along. Many are addicted to alcohol or drugs. Chronic medical problems like diabetes or high blood pressure often have gone either undiagnosed or untreated. Psychiatric problems are rampant.

Many people think that a doctor working in correctional medicine is one who lacks the skills necessary to make it in the "real world." All humility aside, I've found it to be the opposite. "Real world" medicine was a piece of cake.

In my private practice the patients were usually pleasant and motivated. I could get lab tests and x-rays without the hassle of an oversight committee deciding whether it was "medically necessary." I could refer puzzling patients to a specialist colleague without filling out a detailed form trying to justify why I wasn't the guy to take care of that particular problem. Life was good. So why leave this for the wilderness of jails and prisons?

As mentioned, I was burned out. There just didn't seem to be much challenge left, and I didn't look forward to another day at the office. I needed to do something else, tried retirement, failed, and blundered into correctional medicine on the strength of a newspaper ad. It turned out to be something I wished I'd done a decade or two sooner.

Two

On the Job

Las Vegas Avenue, totally misnamed, winds through a decrepit industrial area in the southern suburbs of Colorado Springs. Just before the railroad tracks, a sign directs the curious to the west into the CJC grounds. It's easy to spot because of the Sherman tank squatting opposite the entrance. At first I thought this might be overkill, but closer inspection revealed the tank belonged to the scrap yard next door. I'm pretty sure it's just an ornament.

The driveway snaked past the detox center and the coroner's office before hitting the public parking lot serving the main entrance to the detention center. Inside the main lobby was a window where relatives can post bail for the recently incarcerated. Next to that a flat-screen TV faced a row of chairs where visitors could watch men and women in orange suits stumble through their court appearances.

My trusty '98 Honda motored by the public lot to the official employee lot centered between the south end of the administration building and the evidence building. The 12,000-square-foot evidence building used to be the temporary jail extension housing 200 prisoners when they were building the tower, but now it's just a warehouse.

Lunch, stethoscope, and book in hand, I entered my secret code into the entry pad. I thought "1234" was maybe a little too easy for the pass code, but they probably had people like me in mind when they set it up. Later they changed the entry to a key card, so I didn't have to remember even that much.

Bolted to the side of the building next to the entry is a sturdy-looking tubular structure with a sign saying "Load or Unload Weapons Here." I wasn't sure how the tube was supposed to help you do that, but being unarmed, I let it pass. Maybe you put the muzzle in the opening and blast away until the gun's empty. Unloading your weapon *a la* John Wayne. Whatever.

There weren't any weapons allowed in the jail proper. It's too easy for someone to grab a gun. Pepper spray or a Taser is the limit unless a riot breaks out.

Proceeding past the locker rooms, I entered the main lobby through a side entrance. I was all set to get searched like in all the prisons where I'd worked, but I was ignored at the reception desk. I followed the workers who detoured around the metal detector and buzzed the entrance to the sallyport. I could have carried in a .357.

"Bratzz," the speaker squawked. I figured they were asking for my name or number or something. "Wright. Medical," I said hopefully. The solenoid clicked back.

I proceeded into the port, the heavy metal door clanging shut behind me. Then, nothing. I spied another speaker and button on the far wall. *Surely they know who's in the port*, but I pushed the button anyway.

"Bratzz, Unruch Neebum," the speaker bleated. No clue. The same guy who made the speakers must run a duck farm. I just repeated my name and destination on the hunch that's what they were looking for. The inner door buzzed open.

The inner corridor of CJC would make a terrific bowling alley or maybe, without the roof, a landing strip. Over a hundred yards long and straight as an arrow, it led back to the laundry, snack bar, kitchen and the medical clinic. Entrances to the housing pods peeled off at intervals to the left.

Silent lines of prisoners, handcuffed behind their backs, walked single-file flanked by deputy escorts. The deputies nodded courteously, but otherwise nobody seemed all that excited to see the new doctor.

The medical unit was, to be gracious, utilitarian. A short corridor past medical records led to the nursing station. Wendy and Denise had offices that sandwiched a couple of exam rooms. The doctor's office was…nowhere. I didn't have one.

Wendy said I could have the office down the corridor past where the mental health staff hung out. Just beyond that a room filled with obsolete computer equipment had a desk and chair. Apparently the previous doctor liked to hide out there and do online shopping.

Since being in Siberia wouldn't let me mix with the medical staff and see patients easily, I took one of the exam rooms for my office. Cramped, ugly and noisy, the office also served as the lab for drawing blood and home for the medical assistant. I stole the most comfortable chair I could find, put my art on the walls and settled in.

The internet connection was the saving grace for CJC. In prisons run by the Department of Corrections (DOC), the computer system was so slow and access so restricted that it was easier to bring a book and look information up that way.

At CJC I finally had a real connection. I can't work without some music in the background, so instead of bringing in a stack of CDs, I could fire up Pandora or Jango and actually listen to streaming music all day. Was it okay to do this with their precious bandwidth? I didn't ask.

I made it a point to have soothing music going. No rap, no rock-'n-roll, no heavy metal. Indeed, no vocal music. It's either light classical, solo instrumental, or some flavor of New Age. About 20 percent of my patients remarked that they enjoyed coming to medical because the music made them feel so much better. Probably an equal number hated it. Too bad, worked for me.

Since I went into correctional medicine nine years ago, I'd never had a medical assistant. The nurses, physician assistants, and nurse practitioners all were a great help, but they had schedules and duties all their own, leaving me to muddle through solo. My luck changed at the jail.

Stacy, my medical assistant, was the Radar O'Reilly of CJC. She knew all the prisoners, knew how to flash navigate the electronic medical records system, knew where the supplies were hidden, and knew how to head 'em up and move 'em out in the clinic patient flow. That she owned a liquor store on the side was the cherry on top. You can't get much better than that.

One of the reasons they fired the previous doctor: she was *sooooo slooooowwww*. Lots of ordinary medical procedures she wouldn't do at all, and when she wasn't online doing personal business she saw so few patients that appointments for the clinic were backed up for months.

I'm reasonably quick seeing patients. Patients request a medical appointment by sending a short written request called a kite. The trick is to stay on track by addressing the issue raised by the kite and to not wander around in the eleven other things they think of spontaneously during the visit.

A medical appointment at CJC cost three bucks, and prisoners milked it for everything they could. What they're supposed to do is send a kite on one single issue they want addressed. If they have another problem, they're to send another kite to be addressed at a separate visit.

In theory it seems more efficient to tackle all the problems at once rather than have the patient return for another appointment. What this means in practice is that I'd be sitting there listening to an avalanche of complaints covering everything from warts to cancer. Most will be of minor importance or just fishing expeditions to see if I'd cough up an extra mattress or pain pills. They all take time, so I didn't do it. One visit, one issue. It's amazing how many complaints disappeared when the prisoner had to pay another three bucks to have them addressed.

In their defense I'll admit that the prisoners' trip to medical wasn't all moonlight and roses. Remember the escorted lines of prisoners I passed in the hall on the way in? They're going someplace all in a bunch. That's how they got to medical.

Depending on the demand from a specific housing pod there might be more than a dozen waiting in a common holding cell to see me. On top of that, dental and mental health patients occupied the same space. It made for long waits to see me, and afterward they went to another holding cell to wait until a batch could troop back upstairs.

In other prisons I usually saw about twenty patients per day, but Stacy greeted me every day with a list of forty. "You can do it, Doc," she'd chirp. And I did, but only because there was a high rate of prisoners refusing to come to their medical appointments.

I could understand blowing off an appointment that's been set up by the rules of the facility. We automatically made appointments for patients with diabetes, seizures, high blood pressure and the like. I saw patients with these issues, called chronic care illnesses, for free. Many of my potential patients didn't care about that stuff and didn't want to be bothered to make the trip to medical.

The odd thing was receiving a kite pleading for urgent medical care and then noting a refusal of the kite's author to come to his appointment. This sounds like it should be an anomaly, but I routinely had almost half of my schedule wiped out like this.

I worked with Gloria, a nurse practitioner. She was smart but really, really, really thorough. Gloria needed to gather every scrap of information about her patients. Parental illnesses, travel plans, past lives, Gloria duly recorded everything dribbling from her patients' mouths.

Gloria wasn't lazy, she was just afraid to pull the trigger, make a diagnosis and start a treatment plan. I tried every confidence-building trick I knew, but it just didn't take. Several times a day she'd poke her head around our common wall and say, "Doctor Wright, would you take a look at this?"

I'd put my typing on hold and segue to Gloria's office. "What you got, Gloria?" On this particular day she had Joshua Reynolds with a red lump on his arm.

"Mr. Reynolds has had this sore on his arm for about a week. What do you think?"

Mr. Reynolds was fresh from detox and had a lemon-sized abscess percolating on his arm from his needle use. "Sort of looks like an abscess to me, Gloria."

"I thought so."

"Good call," I said encouragingly.

"Maybe it needs to be drained."

"Probably does."

"Could be MRSA."

"Yep." MRSA is a type of infection caused by bacteria that are resistant to many ordinary antibiotics.

"You want to do it?"

"I can, but you need to learn to do this stuff. I'll watch."

Gloria paled. "Okay, sure…"

"I'll be next door. Give me a shout when you're ready."

I saw two more patients and began to wonder what had happened to Gloria. I peeked around the corner. "Hey, Gloria, how's it going?"

She was knee-deep in sterile gowns, gloves and drapes. It looked like she was prepping for open-heart surgery. Mr. Reynolds had dozed off. "Almost ready," she said.

An abscess is a pocket of pus under the skin, and by definition draining one isn't a sterile procedure. My usual treatment is to clean off the skin, anesthetize a small area and stick a knife in it. I get a culture of the pus that comes out in case I pick the wrong antibiotic, and I'm done in about three minutes start to finish. Gloria was turning this into an epic.

I felt reluctant to criticize. After all, it was her patient and her procedure. What she was doing wasn't wrong, it just wasn't necessary. She was shooting a flea with a cannon. Still, I wanted her to be able to pull the trigger on something, even a cannon.

"Ready to roll?" I said.

She looked at me, resplendent in her sterile gown, gloves, and mask, eyes big as fried eggs, hand trembling slightly with a syringe full of lidocaine.

"Go for it," I prompted.

She started injecting the anesthetic, but the abscess was so ripe it started to leak purulent material through the needle holes. She kept injecting in a circle around the top of the abscess.

"Looks like you've got it surrounded," I said, hoping to get to the actual incision before it all drained through her anesthesia holes.

"Right." She took the scalpel and poised, hesitating above the skin like she was about to harpoon a baby seal.

"It won't take much," I said, hoping to end the suspense.

"Right." She made a scratch with the scalpel, drawing a faint line of blood.

"Maybe a little more than that," I said.

"Right." She advanced the blade through the skin. Pus erupted onto her sterile field.

"Bingo," I said. "Don't forget to catch a culture."

"Right." She looked up again, sweat beaded on her forehead. "Thanks for the help, Doctor Wright."

"Another triumph over the forces of darkness, Gloria."

THREE

THE PATIENTS

I'd been running prison medical clinics for a long time and felt pretty smug about tackling the jail clinic. Are you hearing that "pride before a fall" thing creeping up?

In a prison clinic I sat down with a patient complete with his chart detailing his illnesses and current medications. I usually had notes from providers he'd previously seen detailing their impressions of what was wrong and what the plan was for treatment.

At CJC the patient that sat before me today had slept under a bridge last night. Medical records? Not happening. Medication lists? You wish. Treatment plans? It is to laugh.

I did have Stacy, my medical assistant and the repository of all patient knowledge. Since repeat offenders were so common, she could often tell me what their problems were and what kind of general program they followed during their last incarceration. Huge help. Huge.

My patients at CJC were incredible reservoirs of chronic neglect. I had homeless men whose socks had literally grown into their feet. Women would come in with tampons that had been in place for months.

Hygiene of all sorts was a major issue. I'm blessed with a poor sense of smell, but the stench of some of my patients crossed over to the other senses. It's pretty bad when you can actually see an odor. I won't get into taste.

Like preserving geologic strata, some seemed perversely possessive of their layers of filth. Getting some of the homeless guys into a shower was a major undertaking. Maybe they'd seen *The Wizard of Oz* and thought they'd melt. They'd certainly lose weight. The nurses would sometimes have to hold a man under the stream of water and soap him down like Mom used to do.

Even though I'm not a dentist, I saw dental issues every day. One woman had a horrible layer of candida, a yeast infection, coating her mouth underneath dentures that hadn't been removed in six months. Another man put a layer of bologna on top of his dentures instead of having to purchase denture adhesive. Many patients had dentures picked up at flea markets. These caused lots of ulcers, and they clacked like castanets.

I saw multiple women with no upper front teeth. They told me they got a higher price for oral sex that way. Free enterprise is wonderful.

The prisoners were generally more concerned with getting out of jail than they were about their cholesterol levels. Jail is usually a short-term deal, with the average CJC stay being twenty-seven days. Frequently patients would bond out and only be in jail for a day or two.

While this might sound like a good thing, from a medical point of view it made taking care of patients much tougher. By the time I figured out what the problems were and if any medications or other treatment was involved, the patient might be on his way to Poughkeepsie.

If I was lucky there would be records of prior treatments in the electronic medical records system. If unlucky, I could ask the patient.

Edward McWilliams, a homeless alcoholic in jail for petty larceny, was a case in point:

"So, Mr. McWilliams, I see on your intake form that you have diabetes."

"Yeah."

"Do you take any medication for that?"

"Sometimes."

"Sometimes? What do you take sometimes?"

"That green pill."

"Can you think of a name for that green pill?"

"No."

" Metformin maybe?"

"Yeah, that might be it."

"How often do you take it?"

"Sometimes."

"Once a day? Once a week? Groundhog Day?"

"Once a day if I got it. Shit's expensive."

"When's the last time you took it?"

"Couple of weeks ago. Can't remember exactly."

Stacy had alertly gotten a finger-stick blood sugar when Edward showed up. She handed me the slip.

"Looks like your sugar's a little high today. Take any insulin along with this?"

"Sometimes when I go to the emergency room."

"Well we'll get things rolling now. I'm going to start this twice a day for you. Okay?"

"Sure."

After going over Edward's scanty history and doing a physical, I could see that his diabetes hadn't been under control for a long time. He was underweight and beginning to lose sensation in his feet. His alcohol diet wasn't helping matters, but going into a sermon about getting off the sauce was not going to be helpful at the moment. Edward was a good candidate for going into withdrawal in the near future, so I put a watch on him for that.

I'd see him back in a few days after his sugars were stabilized a bit better and modify the program to fit. His elevated blood pressure was likely due to getting busted and would return to normal in a few days. I'd be watching that too.

If Edward stayed under my care for long enough, I'd get his blood sugar regulated and get a better handle on how the diabetes was ravaging his body. I'd be able to talk to him about these things, but I had no illusions about my effectiveness.

In all probability Edward would be back on the streets in a short time and regress into the alcohol again. At best I'd put a temporary band-aid on his diabetes, which would soon slough off and be forgotten.

I'd referred Edward back to an outside homeless clinic that was constantly overflowing. For the clinic to work, Edward first had to show up, something that was unlikely to happen.

For one thing, Edward didn't have a car or any friends with cars. He often didn't have any money for public transportation, so the clinic visit went by the wayside. If things got bad, and they frequently did, he could catch a ride to the emergency room with the cops.

While metformin isn't the world's most expensive drug, it isn't cheap either, especially if you have no income. Even if Edward got to the clinic and got a prescription, often there would be no money to spare for the medicine.

At $41 for thirty 500 mg tablets that he needed to take twice a day, he had to come up with $20 a week. If he took 1,000 mg twice daily, a common dosage, he'd be down to a week's worth for the same money. Edward didn't have drug insurance, so he was on the hook for the whole amount unless he could get some from the free clinic or a federal program.

Then he had to remember to take it as prescribed. Often he'd try to stretch out the prescription by taking it less often, thereby reducing any effectiveness it might have.

So when Edward showed up in my clinic, dragging his diabetes behind him, I was less than sanguine about my chances of saving him from continued deterioration. The lengthy discussions I used to have with my private patients were pretty much lost on Edward. He was just getting by the best he can.

On a more positive note, getting busted could often save a life. Unless the offenders were return customers or went to a free clinic and were already following a medical program, I was often the first doctor they'd seen, maybe ever.

Many chronic illnesses like hypertension, elevated cholesterol, diabetes, or thyroid trouble are silent killers. If I could find these and educate the patients enough to get them to continue on a program, I could literally save their lives.

Sadly, many didn't want to be saved. Although I got all kinds coming to the jail, many had the life beaten out of them, and they just didn't care anymore. Getting out of jail and back to their drugs or booze topped the list of things they looked forward to.

I don't say this to be mean-spirited. While the inmates I treated in prisons largely deserved to be there, the jail is a different story. Many of my jail patients weren't nasty, violent people, they're just sad. Life had dealt them a bad hand through parental neglect, childhood abuse, sexual exploitation, limited intelligence, or just plain bad luck.

For sure I saw lots of the other kind who victimize their children or habitually choose the criminal path out of laziness, arrogance, meanness, or greed. Jail is just a way station for these criminals. They'd been there before, and they'd soon be back until they rack up enough points to be sent to prison for an extended stay.

The two classes presented to me very differently. The ones who were headed for prison usually came off as arrogant and demanding. If something wasn't to their liking, it was always someone else's fault.

The other group presented with a kind of acceptance that things just weren't ever going to get better. They're resigned to it and, like someone in a deep depression, they couldn't muster the energy to see out of their hole. They accepted my medical ministrations passively with the attitude that nothing would make much difference in their lives anyway.

It was tough treating chronic diseases if I was the only member of the team. The people I could really help were those who sensed that their lives could be better if they took some initiative themselves. Sometimes I could make that connection, but too often I felt them slipping away, as if I was pulling them up from a well with a greased rope.

It was way different from the private practice I used to know. There, patients would come to me with a problem they wanted fixed. They were motivated and willing to do whatever was required to get better. That's half the battle. If I did my part, thing generally worked out.

When patients refused to come to chronic care clinic or to take critical medications, I had a choice to make. When I work in prisons, the choice is easier. If an inmate has sky-high blood pressure or elevated cholesterol, I call him down to clinic and have a chat.

Sometimes he didn't understand his disease or why he should take medication. That's easily fixed and everybody goes home happy. If he thought he understood the situation but blew it off, that's his privilege. He can refuse medical care as long as he's capable of making rational decisions, even if the decisions are bad ones.

Alonzo Roller, a hard-case 57-year-old white-haired inmate, a repeat offender with high blood pressure, sullenly slouched into my office and sat with one cheek on the exam table and one leg pointed toward the exit. I didn't need a course in reading body language to guess that Alonzo wouldn't be staying long. Still…

"Mr. Roller, I see your blood pressure's been running pretty high. Has anyone talked to you about that?"

"Yeah."

"Blood pressure this high can give you a stroke or a heart attack. Any interest in maybe getting on some medicine to bring it down?"

"Nope."

"Any reason why? It's pretty simple and could tack another ten or twenty years onto your life."

"Fuck you."

Eloquence was not Alonzo's strong suit, but the message was clear enough. I dismissed him with the offer of revisiting the issue in the future if he changed his mind. Inmates like this rarely do.

I'm fine with that. It's his funeral, not mine. As long as I'd done my best to educate him about what was wrong and what the consequences were of taking one course or another, I'd done my job. My personal feelings about whether he's an idiot or not are beside the point.

The magic phrase for knowing when I was talking to one of these guys was, "I know my own body." This meant I was talking to a lump of Jell-O and might as well save my breath. I don't think I've ever converted one of these true believers until he fell over with a stroke or diabetic ketoacidosis.

Now we're down to the group who were just too lazy to get out of bed and take their free government-supplied medication. As long as they'd had one of my come-to-Jesus talks, I had no problem cancelling their prescriptions. Benny Medici was one of these.

"Mr. Medici, I see you've been missing your morning insulin. Any problem with the medication?"

"It's too early, man."

"Diabetes, like the tide, waits for no man."

"What?"

"Just an expression. Look, your sugars are out of sight by noon. Then the nurses give you extra, and sometimes you're crashing in the evening. You've got to take the morning dose."

"I'm a night person, man. I don't get up that early. Can't the nurses come in and wake me up?"

"The nurses are not your mom. Take some responsibility. Get your ass out of bed and get the shot. Simple."

"Yeah, whatever."

You can guess what continues to happen. Putting together a program for inmates that won't take the simplest steps to help themselves is, to put it mildly, challenging.

With most chronic health conditions the consequences of their refusals weren't immediately apparent. What happens with neglected high blood pressure, high cholesterol, or uncontrolled diabetes is irreversible damage down the line, leading to chronic disabilities and shortened lives. Some might think this is a societal benefit, but I can't look at it that way as their physician.

In the jail things were more complicated than they were in prison settings. I couldn't just cut off medications like I could in the penitentiaries. If I had a patient who refused to come to chronic care clinic, I had to bring him down to clinic (no charge) and explain the nature of his disease and the recommended therapy. If he still refused to come, I needed to do the whole process a total of three times before I could discontinue any prescriptions.

This was not only a hassle for me, but the nurses had to get the medication ready, offer it to the patient, get a signed refusal of the medication from him and repeat the process every day until I was allowed to cut it off. Even then I had to offer him the option to resume chronic care every month…forever.

But am I done with it then? Noooo. If the medications are considered "critical" like anti-seizure or diabetic medications, I had to leave them on the books even though the patient continued to refuse them every day.

Maybe other jails are more sensible, but CJC more than bent over backwards to avoid any sliver of appearance that they were neglecting the needs of our inmates. From a corporate standpoint, I suppose it made some kind of cover-your-ass sense, but not for anyone who had to do the actual work.

Another way that prison populations differed from those of the jail was homelessness. At least while they were in prison, inmates had a home, many for the majority of their lives. While maybe not the best situation, it did remove a lot of uncertainty.

The jail, on the other hand, is tasked with housing short-term detainees. No matter what the reason for their incarceration at the jail, the prospect of moving on in the near future created stress and anxiety. Some would go to prison, some to deportation, but many were released either through posting bail or serving out their sentence.

While being released from jail sounds like a good thing, for many of my patients it meant a return to homelessness on the streets without the prospects of food, shelter or medical care. For some, being in jail was the only thing that kept them alive. Indeed, I saw lots of patients caught in the revolving door of arrest, jail, release, and back again just because they had no place else to go.

Henry Bastian was one of these guys. A 56-year-old man who looked 70, Henry presented to my clinic for his intake physical. Reviewing his records I saw a regular stream of arrests about every three months for several years. Although I usually don't inquire into the reasons for my patients' incarceration, I asked Henry why he couldn't stay out of the slammer.

"Doc, I can't make it out there. On the street I'm nothing. In here I'm a king. I been around the block a few times, so I get respect in here, three squares a day and a place to sleep."

The homeless were a mixed lot, but there was a strong streak of mental illness among them. Nearly half of all homeless people have a history of traumatic brain injury. I used to think that this was because of the rough life they encountered on the streets, but I learned that almost all of the initial injuries occurred before they became homeless.

It makes sense that this would be the case. With a head injury a person might be less able to concentrate or focus on their work. Personalities can change, leading to degraded ability to get along in their former social circles. Work suffers and they lose their jobs. Marriages crumble along with family relationships. Finances erode, and a negative spiral culminates with life alone on the streets.

This doesn't mean that these men were brawlers. Nearly half of the brain injuries are related to sports or other recreational activities.

Correctional medicine is a different animal from private medical care. People often came to me because they were required to by the facility rules rather than by any burning desire to improve their health. I not only had to be the diagnostician, but also the cheerleader to generate some motivation in an apathetic patient. Sometimes I saw a spark, and that's what kept me going to the next patient with a little bit of hope.

I burned out of being an ear surgeon because I'd seen it all, or at least thought I had. I think if people burn out in correctional medicine it's because of a feeling of swimming in molasses. The endless tide of new admissions and the inertia of administrators make for professional frustration if you let it get to you. Like molasses, it's sweet for a while, but then things get sticky.

Four

Beauty Tips from the Big House

Just because you're behind bars is no excuse for letting personal appearance slip. Jails have basic hygiene items for sale to inmates, but beyond that it's a crap shoot. Some have limited cosmetic items, but most don't have even that. Time to improvise.

Inmates used makeup for lots of different reasons. Jail isn't conducive to that healthy glow we associate with robust youth, so the most obvious goal was to just look better. Another was merely to look different. Yet another was sheer boredom and the need to shake it up a little.

Females were the greatest practitioners of cosmetology, but males participated too, especially the overtly homosexual crowd. I wondered why the women would go to so much trouble with improvised makeup.

As a male, I'm already branded as clueless when it comes to personal appearance. I'm told, however, that women do this primarily for the benefit of other women. One of the nurses told me that if women were dressing for men, they'd all be naked.

With limited availability of materials but lots of time, the inmates became endlessly inventive. I didn't have much personal experience with these techniques, but the nurses verified what I'd heard, and I'd even seen some confirmed on TV in the *Orange is the New Black* series. Here's a primer on glamour in the slammer.

Want wavy hair? Tampons or pencils serve as hair curlers. Toilet paper cores or even socks will work. In a pinch braid wet hair and let it dry overnight. Would you rather go for the spiked look? Use clear toothpaste for hair gel. Need coloring and gel together? Jelly mixed with cocoa butter to make it not so sticky does the trick and makes you smell and taste better too.

Hair coloring is a snap with Kool-Aid, especially if you don't want to make a long-term commitment. Make sure to use the unsweetened kind to avoid stickiness. Artificial sweeteners can irritate your eyes, so just go plain.

Tropical punch or a mixture of black cherry and strawberry makes a great bright red. Cherry gives a deeper hue. Strawberry with grape results in a more purplish color.

Add a little conditioner to the powder to make a paste and brush it in. Cover with plastic wrap overnight and rinse it with warm water in the morning. Dry, and *voila*! Color that lasts until your next shampoo. If you have some Kool-Aid powder left over, mix it with a little Vaseline to make a phenomenal blush. Works as lipstick too.

If you don't happen to have Kool-Aid, black tea can work wonders to darken hair, especially if you're blonde. Cherry juice works too, but it's hard to find. Anything waxy with color that can be melted down is another option for the color palette. Complete your hairstyle with a ponytail secured with a rubber band extracted from your panties.

If your cellie objects to your bushy eyebrows, he or she can help by teasing them with a pair of strings or rubber bands. I've never seen this done, but sources insist that a skilled operator can pluck out stray hairs this way better than using a pair of tweezers. Where can you get string? That's another use for the multifunctional tampon.

After the eyebrows are reduced, use a Magic Marker for eyeliner or eyebrow pencil. Colored pencils work for this too. Just soak them in water for a couple of minutes to soften the lead. This works for lip liner too. Tar from window seals makes acceptable mascara or eyeliner.

Silver glitter from greeting cards becomes eye shadow. A paste of baby powder and coffee grounds is good if you don't want to be as flamboyant. Apply it with a thin coating of Vaseline to make it stay in place longer. Want some color? M&Ms can serve here, or grab the comics from the Sunday paper and dissolve some of that ink to use. Ink from a regular ballpoint pen can serve as eyeliner or mascara.

If the Kool-Aid lipstick isn't cutting it, try stain from cherries or beets. Careful, they can really stain skin on other parts of the body, and you'll never get it out of your prison uniform. In a pinch, Jolly Rancher candies can substitute for other sources of color. Chapped lips from licking the Jolly Rancher lipstick? Apply some shaving gel.

If you've had a long night and wake up to those bags under your eyes, grab some Preparation H and banish them. I hear denture cream works as well.

To tighten up that slack skin have your Mexican buddy chew up some hot peppers and mix it with Shea cocoa butter. The peppers contain capsaicin, the same chemical that's in pepper spray, but I'm told this paste doesn't burn the skin. I think I'll pass on this one.

If you've got an orange, the inside of the peel rubbed on cheeks will close pores, tighten the skin and make it look smoother. Wait, don't throw it away yet. The outside of the peel has the vitamin C that works wonders on crow's feet or other wrinkles around the eyes.

Got a hot date or a parole hearing and your face looks like a mine field? Clear those zits with an aspirin paste or a dab of toothpaste.

Teeth dull? Strawberries can whiten them. Using salt, preferably with some baking soda, as a substitute for toothpaste is great. The tiny crystals scour as well as any paste.

Unsightly nails? If you can score some fine sandpaper, you're in business.

For smoothing the rough skin on your feet, try the deodorant stick supplied for indigent prisoners.

For a finishing touch, apply perfume from a scratch-and-sniff ad in a magazine. You can also harken back to the original perfumers and use flowers for their fragrant oils.

No outfit is complete without jewelry. Here's where a combination of artistry and infinite time combine to produce some amazing pieces. Toilet paper is the substrate for remarkable creations ranging from detailed model airplanes and delicate roses (some are on display in the CJC lobby), to personal adornments. Inmates weave beautiful crucifixes and necklaces from thin strips of plastic garbage bags or string. Intricate soap art is almost a prison cliché.

FIVE

KITES

In the jail we couldn't have the prisoners wandering around and dropping into medical whenever they felt like it. The kite system of sending a short note to medical requesting an appointment was common to both the jail and Colorado prisons.

Unless the prisoner writes really, really small a kite had space for only a couple of sentences about why he wanted to be seen. From the prisoner's standpoint, his kite had multiple functions, and it was as carefully crafted as a haiku.

The best of all possible outcomes of sending a kite was to receive free medical care without having to actually appear in the medical clinic. Here's one from Alan Waymen, a forger looking down the barrel of being a three-time loser:

I've been seen for the same thing three times already. I just need a refill on my muscle relaxers. Nothing's changed. No need for an appointment. Thank you.

Alan's probably right that nothing has changed. What hasn't changed is his ability to con providers in whatever facility he came from. Muscle relaxants like Baclofen or Flexeril are of limited utility at best and are rarely useful beyond a week or two. What they are is sedatives closely related to antidepressants. Prisoners love that, but from a medical standpoint they're fairly worthless.

Alan doesn't want to get into a big discussion about this. He just wants his ticket punched and another truckload of Flexeril delivered to his doorstep without a lot of fuss. Notice that the kite has the feeling of "These aren't the droids you're looking for."

So the wording of the kite emphasizes that (1) the problem has already been exhaustively evaluated; (2) several prescriptions for this have already been written by other providers, subtly implying that I should get on the bandwagon; (3) the condition is stable with the implication that the medication is effective in treating the problem, and (4) re-evaluating the situation would just be a waste of everyone's time. Like many kites, it ends with an ingratiating "Thank you."

The bonuses for Alan if this rides through is that he won't have to come to medical, wait for a long time to be seen and taken back, take a chance that he'll say the wrong thing and get his request denied, and he'll save three bucks. A trifecta.

The penultimate-worst case for Alan is if I send back the kite with a time for a medical appointment to discuss the issue. If the present prescription has some time to run, Alan won't show, afraid that it might be cancelled. He's hoping that I'll forget the whole thing, and he's probably got a good bet there unless he pisses me off somehow, and I take the time to review his medications in a free moment. Not likely to happen. I've got 1,499 other mouths to feed.

The worst case is if I insist on an appointment with the provision that if he doesn't show up, I'll discontinue the prescription. He knows he's screwed either way. Sending a kite is always rolling the dice, and it's often better to let sleeping dogs lie.

Another kite came from an inmate who wanted his name copyrighted. He figured that if nobody could use his name without his written permission then he would be exempt from disciplinary write-ups and other jail unpleasantries.

I tried to tell him that while it might work for The Artist Formerly Known as Prince, it wasn't going to work for him. He carried the grievance all the way to a formal lawsuit. I kind of lost track after that, but in America anything is possible.

I keep a file of some of my more entertaining and gross kites. Since you asked (punctuation and spelling mostly intact):

I really need to see the obstetrician as soon as possible. My eyes and my glasses I have now are not in good shape.

I am having a metal/puss taste coming from my throt & got white chunks coming fron tonsils.

I went to the school of education and hard knocks.

As of Tuesday I will have absolutely no teeth left as there gonna take them all out could you please talk to kitchen and get set for a soft diet and I truly wouldn't mind peanut butter and jelly sandwhiches as often as possible all the time would be cool as theres a lot or protein and I could eat this okay.

Would like glass's cuz I need them

I would like a STD test done please and thank you, Also I have these weird bumps down by me penis I would like to know what they are because there freaking me out.

I am on the top bunk and I feel that I am too heavy for it. I tried to move to the bottom bunk with no relief.

I am requesting some denture. I have been without for almost 2 ½ year now and I am missing out on a lot of good food.

I was wondering if I were to be tested for any and all S.T.D.'s, to include H.I.V., Hep C, how long would it be before I take this test and how long before the result? Schedule Me!!

I have some kind of rash on my face. Ive never had it until I got to this place.

I'm not taking any more medications. I don't need to be a test dummy of these weird medications. I was doing just fine before I came here.

Request of T.B test and copy of result to check into Homeless Shelter. TB test copy is required by shelter for bed space.

Still having chronic lower back pain, and also Involuntary muscle stiches, and tingling up and down left arm, numbness in finger tips.

I am anemic I need iron pill, Ensure shake daily or I will faint and dry skin cream and coltar shampoo

I need some Neospermia for a cut on my hand.

I'd like to get an appotomical exam.

The kites were a great preview of the encounter to come, but not always. Evin Nicholas, a frequent flier with a penchant for petty theft, sent me this one:

Pain in left knee for weeks. Terrible. Can't sleep. Please see ASAP

This seemed fairly straightforward, but when Evin showed up for his appointment, it was a different story.

"So, Mr. Nicholas, what's going on?" I'd learned to never suggest an ailment or symptom to a patient. Let them come to me.

"I got terrible gas, Doc. You gotta give me something."

Right then I knew the knee complaint was bogus. By not specifically asking about his kite, I'd put the onus on him to remember why he asked to be seen in the first place. It was a good indication of how important the problem was or if it existed at all. Now I could address the gas problem and pretty much ignore the knee kite unless he happened to remember his terrible pain and bring it up.

What happened to the terrible knee pain? My best guess is it didn't exist in the first place. Evin was likely sitting around after playing a round of basketball and noticed some soreness in his joints. He reflexively grabbed a kite and scribbled off a request, thinking that maybe I would rush up with some ibuprofen and a cold drink. With the attention span of a fruit fly, Evin then went on to the next diversion. Just a guess.

Kites could be moving targets. Even though I could see patients pretty promptly after they sent their kites, their presentation at the time of appointment could be totally different. Take Mr. Madden, a 5'-10", 300-pound lump who kited for "Total body pain."

When I saw him the next day, the pain had morphed into horrible, terrible, excruciating foot pain. Even I felt sorry for his feet having to carry that mass around. Nonetheless, I checked a uric acid as gout was a possibility.

When Madden came back two days later for follow-up, I found the uric acid was indeed elevated and started to explain this to him. Apparently feeling that all this technical mumbo-jumbo wasn't going to score him any narcotics, he spontaneously mentioned that his arms were paralyzed.

"Really?" I asked.

"Just happened this morning, Doc."

"They seemed to be working okay when you walked in."

He twisted his torso around and let his left arm flop on my desk. He looked at me expectantly.

"Pretty amazing," I said. "We'd better look into this."

The solution, as I'll detail later, was to place Mr. Madden in Cell One, a time-out sort of place with a central drain and no furnishings. Time passed. I called him back in.

This time he struggled into the office with a kind of Quasimodo-on-a-bad-day stumbling shuffle, arms flailing at his sides like clumps of seaweed, his neck cocked at a tortuous 30° angle.

"All fixed?" I asked.

"Worse, Doc," he mumbled, lurching into a chair. "Paralyzed in my legs too."

"Moved down, eh?" I observed. He nodded sadly.

"Pain too?"

"Horrible. All over."

I couldn't continue. "Mr. Madden, this has to be the worst performance I've ever witnessed. You're not getting anything from me today. Come back when the paralysis clears up, and we'll talk about the gout."

"I need to go to the hospital. I need—"

"Nothing. Nada. Out."

Scowling, he contorted himself upright and shambled toward the waiting room.

Quasimodo, besides the giant wart over his eye, had Esmeralda. Madden had someone even more compelling. Not an hour later, Denise, our Director of Nursing, got a call from Madden's mother giving everyone hell for neglecting (deliberately and indifferently) her precious son. Denise poked her head in my office, a questioning look on her face.

I shook my head. "You wouldn't believe it if I told you," I said. "Have him sign a release of information form so we can talk to her." Due to all the privacy regulations, we couldn't tell anybody anything without written permission.

Denise had Madden sign the release form with his totally paralyzed hand. At least he didn't think to drool on the form. Denise, more diplomatic than I, chatted with his mom, giving her a somewhat different version of the encounter than her son had told her. Mom was mollified. Madden spontaneously recovered sometime during the next twenty-four hours. Crisis averted. A day in the life.

Like kites, grievances are written communication with medical, but with more room on the form to expound. You haven't experienced eye strain until you've tried to decipher an entire page filled with misspelled sentence fragments written with a blunt black Sharpie.

Dr. Writhght has told me that he is not a certified neurologist and has refused proper medical treatment an CHC medical has denied me a neurologist that can give me not only proper care but tell who ever is in charge like commander potlatch to move me to place less stressfull then medical or C2. If you need my attorney # let me know.

Well, I was all over this one, although I'd never seen my name mangled so thoroughly. The deputies told me that Mr. Lockley, the author of this tome, had encountered some of his former associates on the housing pod. The reunion was apparently not pleasant, and Lockley wanted out of there before he became a casualty. He thought that getting a medical transfer out was his best ticket.

CJC takes care to separate potential sources of trouble like this, but we have to know about them before we can do anything. If Lockley decided not to say anything on intake and he wasn't known to the personnel, he might end up in the wrong pod.

I was taken to the doctor and told about treatment for Hep C. I would like my $8 back. I'm not sure but that fits the description of extortion or theft.

I'm reluctant to argue with experts on extortion and theft, but I still think three bucks for a doctor's visit is a good deal. I wasn't sure what the other five dollars was about.

I have yet to receive a response to the kite I sent in regards to the $7.00 that I paid for visit that never happen. I was not in CJC on 7/29/11. I was at Memorial giving birth so I would like my money back.

Hey, I don't know if it's true, but it's the best excuse I've heard today.

I sent a kite for a medical appointment. Please do not charge me any money for this I need it for food.

I'll have to remember this one the next time I make an appointment with my doctor.

Im just inquiring if Im gunna be reimbursed for the 4 days that my shampoo wasn't on the med cart or it might have been 3 days.

Well, gee. And the masseuse didn't show either.

Then there were the jailhouse lawyers with typical tough guy language. The following grievance began with this as the bolded heading:

Medical Grievance for non-mental Health treatment, towit a deliberate indifference to me serious medical need.

Of course, he went on to grieve not being able to see a psychiatrist right away for his non-mental health complaints, but he had a couple of the buzz words in there "deliberate indifference" and "serious medical need." I think they copied these from an old Americans with Disabilities Act publication. The ADA is the act that guarantees equal access to persons with disabilities. Prisoners love it. He managed to stick "towit" in there too. Haven't seen that in a while. Nice.

I couldn't help it. I overheard the nurse midwife in the next room doing a pelvic exam and questioning a newly admitted patient who complained of vaginal discharge.

"Are you sexually active?"

"No, I mostly just lies there."

This woman was not sharp enough to memorize jokes or come up with her own snappy quips. Really. I am not making this up.

What happened when a pregnant woman got busted? It wasn't unusual. About 6 percent of women are pregnant when arrested. If she knows she's pregnant—and many don't, almost to the time they deliver—she's put on a prenatal diet and scheduled to see the nurse midwife, who comes by every two weeks. She's scheduled to be seen on a regular basis by the midwife, but it's common for the appointments to be refused.

It's was hard to know why they refused, but a couple of things came into play. Some were just too lazy. I saw it all the time in medical clinic, and it seemed to carry over into OB appointments. Some women seemed to dissociate from their pregnancy, willing it to go away. For others it was a reminder of their pregnant condition and that they were in jail. All these things conspired to keep some women from getting the prenatal care they and their babies needed.

At CJC all new female arrivals got a pregnancy test to sort things out. We didn't take their word for it one way or the other. Never can tell when an immaculate conception might occur.

Some women claimed to be pregnant, thinking it would get them a lower bail amount, help them with sympathy during their court appearance, or just score better food. The pre-natal diet is higher in calcium and vitamins than the regular fare.

The mom-to-be was housed in general population in a lower bunk. Among the other women she could often get some facts-of-life info that she'd been missing up to that point. Pregnancy complicated an already scary time adjusting to the chaos of jail with the crowding and constant yelling. Just getting used to the smells of confined humanity could be a major hurdle.

When she was ready to deliver it's off to the hospital, accompanied by a deputy. Just like any other woman, she had a choice of natural childbirth or drug-assisted. Contrary to what you might think, more went the natural route.

In Colorado she can't keep the baby in jail, so the tyke goes to family, adoption, or Children's Protective Services. It was especially sad when this was the sixth or seventh child, and the mother couldn't remember the names or ages of her other kids.

Frequently there was a history of sexual abuse since an early age, or prostitution. The mother may have had no clue about who the father might be. Sometimes we needed to wait and see what the race of the baby was before the field was narrowed. Abused women with a non-violent crime history might qualify for family-based treatment programs as an alternative to incarceration.

If the woman was addicted to narcotics, we kept her in the medical clinic and continued the drugs. If she went off them, there was a good chance the withdrawal would kill the baby. The baby was born addicted to the drug and needed to be treated for withdrawal. Welcome to the world. Quitting cold turkey is something addicted women sometimes tried when they found out they were pregnant, usually with fatal consequences for the unborn child.

When it was time for the delivery, the inmate rode to the hospital by ambulance. More painful than the birth was the new mother's realization that she wouldn't see her baby again until she got out of jail. She had two days to memorize the little face, to kiss and hug the new arrival, to try to squeeze a lifetime of bonding into forty-eight hours. It wasn't enough, of course, and the return to jail was wrenching for everyone.

SIX

THE SYSTEM

Although it's hard to be exact, jails go back a long way. The Greeks used them when citizens couldn't pay fines. The Romans were the first to use jails as punishment rather than simply for detention. In the Middle Ages the ability to have someone imprisoned or killed was a measure of a person's power and authority.

This was not without backlash. In the eighteenth century people began to chafe at summary executions and torture. Authorities, sensitive to their public images, saw imprisonment as a workable alternative to more violent means of controlling unruly citizens. At the same time, a movement arose advocating prisons as places of rehabilitation where prisoners could be instructed in correct behavior.

With the underlying ethic of "Out of sight, out of mind," many European nations simply shipped prisoners away to penal colonies as an alternative to the liberally dispensed death penalty. They sent masses of prisoners to infamous destinations such as Devil's Island in French Guiana, Siberia, Australia, or even Louisiana, presumably prior to Mardi Gras.

Sometimes authorities did away with the necessity of transportation entirely, confining prisoners to old stationary sailing ships called, appropriately, hulks. While prisons migrated to land and became larger state-run facilities, jails continued to be local affairs intended for short-term detention. Here, prisoners could be held awaiting trial or for short sentences imposed by the court. CJC is such a facility serving El Paso County, home to Colorado Springs.

Granted that jailing people has been going on for a while, but why do we do it at all? There are several schools of thought about that.

At first blush, we put people in jail to punish them. Jails and prisons are unpleasant places, and being sentenced to spend time there carries a social stigma beyond the time spent behind bars.

Besides punishment, it sounds reasonable that the unpleasant nature of incarceration would act as a deterrent to people doing things that would land them there. Deterrence has two assumptions. First, if a person spends time in jail, he'll be deterred from committing a crime that would return him to that situation. Second, fear of similar punishment will deter others from criminal acts.

Both of these assumptions have supporters and detractors in different studies. It seems that the severity of the punishment doesn't have much effect on deterrence, but the certainty of punishment does. After all, if you don't think you're going to get caught, the penalty is really beside the point.

The time spent in prison can be an opportunity for rehabilitation, but it is more certainly a time of incapacitation. This simply means that while a person is in jail, he doesn't have the opportunity to commit further crimes. This was the overriding principle behind the creation of maximum-security prisons like Alcatraz. There was little thought that the prisoners housed within would become model citizens. They were there simply to get them off the streets for extended periods of time.

Even the subject of rehabilitation is conflicted. One school looks at jail time as "schools of crime" where association with other criminals increases the probability of returning to criminal activity when released. Another sees incarceration as an opportunity for retraining and reeducation in adopting a different lifestyle.

While the American model yields fairly dismal results in terms of rehabilitation, the model followed in Scandinavia is much more salutary. I'll talk about that in a later chapter.

I'd never known the difference between the sheriff's office and the police department. I was soon educated that the police department serves the incorporated limits of Colorado Springs, while the sheriff is responsible for the rest of the county. Dispatchers route 911 calls to the agency responsible for the area of the call.

The sheriff in Colorado Springs is also the fire warden for prairie and forest fires. This might seem like a Mickey Mouse type of job, but in the Springs it's a big deal.

Two summers ago the Waldo Canyon fire made national news, eventually covering almost thirty square miles in the Pike National Forest just west of town. Driven by high winds, it roared down the Front Range Mountains to destroy almost 350 homes in the Colorado Springs suburbs and threaten the

Air Force Academy. I had my bags packed and ready to go as the fire tried to jump I-25 into Colorado Springs proper.

Waldo Canyon was the most destructive fire in Colorado history in terms of property lost until last summer, when the Black Forest, a community sheltered in pine trees just east of Colorado Springs proper, erupted in flames. Tinder-dry undergrowth and high winds drove the fire to destroy over 500 homes. Again, everyone in Colorado Springs was poised to flee depending on which way the wind blew the fire.

Both fires are believed to be arson, so the sheriff would be involved even if he wasn't the fire warden. He did get a lot of TV face time and for reasons unknown got into a very public pissing contest with the Black Forest fire chief. Politics is never far away from the sheriff's office. More about that later.

On a more traditional law-enforcement note a couple dozen people were arrested during and after the fires for looting the evacuated homes and stealing materials brought in to rebuild them.

The sheriff has the job of administering the jail, but since activities like food or medical services aren't really in his line, he hires outside contractors to do these chores. Correctional Healthcare Companies, a huge company based in Colorado, got the job for CJC. So when I came to work at the jail, I wasn't working for the sheriff; I was working for the corporation that had the contract. This, I would learn, was a fatal flaw.

Seven

Protocols

Clinical protocols, printed step-by-step outlines of how to handle a situation, seem like a good idea. They're designed to ensure that you won't forget a critical item, at the same time relieving you of the necessity to think about what you're doing.

Jails are big on protocols because staff may be inexperienced in coping with common problems. Jails have a big staff turnover, which guarantees the greenhorns will be on duty at night. A protocol prevents unnecessary calls to the higher-ups for guidance, especially since the higher-ups may have forgotten how to manage the problem anyway.

I'm all for protocols that prevent nurses calling me in the middle of the night. I personally would not want to be on the receiving end of medical advice issued by a semi-comatose doctor at 3 a.m. The nurses know this is often a counterproductive exercise as well, leading to confused orders and a grumpy doctor. Better to fall back on a protocol and leave the details to business hours.

I drew the line when the protocols applied to me. While this may sound elitist, I'm prepared to come to my own defense. CJC had a good EMR (electronic medical records) system. By this I mean that, unlike the EMR system in the Department of Corrections, it can put letters on the screen as fast as I can type.

For those of you with a real computer this might not seem like a big deal. Try to hold your concentration when your typing doesn't show up on the screen for twenty or thirty seconds. Then the letters stagger one at a time across the screen like arthritic ants crawling through superglue. It's a government system. Nobody's in a hurry. Compared to DOC, the jail's computer system is a gazelle.

Part of CJC's system is a series of protocols that are supposed to be used to enter data at every patient visit. Sounds good so far, doesn't it? Just fill in the blanks. Except that a committee got hold of each disease description and put an item for every single conceivable rat fact that could possibly be associated with the illness. And there's a separate protocol for each and every complaint the offender might come up with. So…

Would you rather type in a short description of the pertinent facts of the visit or fill out several pages of checkboxes and blanks covering information that isn't even remotely pertinent to the current transaction with your patient? And on the next visit would you rather paw through pages of extraneous information or just read a short paragraph or two. Hmm? I thought so. Me too.

This precipitated my first run-in with the Cheeses at corporate. They'd spent lots of money and committee meetings putting these forms together and by gum I was going to use them. Or else.

"Or else what?" I asked via email.

Apparently they hadn't considered this option too carefully. They'd been looking for a doctor replacement for the better part of a year, and there wasn't a line forming outside to apply. I was granted permission to use a "modified protocol form," which turned out to be a blank page. Super. I'm in.

They also shot back that if I would care to modify the protocols (chuckle) on my own, they'd be pleased to consider changing them (guffaw). I thought, *what the hell,* and took a half-dozen of the most egregious offerings on hypertension, seizures, cholesterol and such. I rewrote them, taking each down to a single page. Off they went to the Cheeses. It seems that they're still in committee, as I haven't received an answer in almost a year.

The trouble with protocols is they are made by people who don't have to use them. Take high blood pressure, for instance. In a chronic care clinic visit I've got maybe ten minutes to establish some kind of rapport with my patient, take a history along with reviewing whatever old information I might have, do a physical, determine the diagnosis, formulate a treatment plan, and communicate the plan to the patient, hopefully with some buy-in on his side.

Unless I'm dealing with some exotic cause of the hypertension, I don't need much info. What have his blood pressures been running? Is he taking any medications? Any salient physical findings? Does he want the blood pressure problem treated (many don't)?

After this, I'm gilding the lily with information that might be interesting, but is usually extraneous. Remember, my goal is to keep this guy alive and point him on a path to getting better in the future. I'm not writing research papers here.

The protocol wants me to list all family members with any kind of cardiovascular disease. Is this relevant information? Yes. Is it important to our current goal? No.

"Is there anybody else in your family with high blood pressure?"

Potential answers:

"I dunno."

"I think my uncle took some medicine for something."

"My brother has high blood pressure." (He's adopted.)

"Yeah, my mother used to have it." (Great. Too bad I'm not treating your mom.)

While entertaining to reminisce about family illnesses, they usually don't have much to add when I'm coming up with a treatment plan. I can see the problem sitting here in front of me whistling Dixie through his meth-ravaged teeth. Filling out a family tree takes time I don't have for a payoff that's at best marginal.

I'm aware that all my old professors at University of Michigan Medical School would roll over in their collective graves to hear me say it, but I don't have time or resources for the million-dollar workup. An old medical maxim that "Common things are common," applies here. If I can get something reasonable started on a hundred patients, I'll worry later about the five that didn't respond like I thought they would.

Ideally, I'd have the offenders fill out their own medical history sheet like you do when you go to visit a doctor. I'd scan down the sheet, pick out the "Yes" answers, decide if it's anything to even ask about, and move on. Quick and efficient. Unfortunately, this option does not apply here.

For the most part, my jail patients don't know their medical histories. They're not even sure what substances they shot into their veins last night. If I gave a roomful of offenders a three-page medical questionnaire to fill out before seeing me, I'd come back to a roomful of paper airplanes and graffiti.

Then there's the drug thing. "Are you taking any medications?" brings out a cornucopia of replies.

"Yeah, I used to take some stuff."

"I use my sister's meds."

"I just take what they give me at the clinic."

"Yeah, I take 400 units of Lantus (a type of insulin)." This would be a lethal dose. Closer questioning reveals he might take 40 units of Lantus when he has the money. Pesky decimal points.

Asking about medications provides a great opportunity for obfuscation.

"You can check my meds at Walgreens. I'm not sure which one. I use three or four of 'em. You could check at Wal-Mart too. I get some there. And the VA in Oklahoma."

"Yeah, they got me on MS Contin (morphine) and Percocets (a narcotic) for my back." Some of them might find a doctor to actually do this, but most likely they're talking about what they got from the ER doctor last time they were there, a one-time dose to move them out the door.

"My doctor said I need to stay on Vicodin (another narcotic) for these stomach pains." Really? Which doctor?

"Dr. Singh in Kuala Limpur."

"Dr. Andrews, but he retired right after I saw him."

"Dr. Abrams, but the clinic where he worked burned down."

"I forget his name, but he worked at a hospital in Idaho. It's a big hospital on a corner."

So the protocols with their neat boxes aren't much help in the wild and wooly reaches of jail medicine. I think checklists (one page or less, please) of things to remember are great and don't consume much in the way of time or resources. As the years advance I'm grateful for anything that will keep me from blundering too badly. Just don't pretend that multiple sheets of fill-in-the-blanks are an effective substitute for critical thinking.

EIGHT

BUSTED

Police can arrest someone if (1) they see him breaking any law; (2) they have "probable cause" to believe he committed a felony; or (3) they have a warrant for his arrest. My patients often made the mistake of arguing their innocence with the arresting officer. They should have saved their breath. Guilt or innocence is not up to the police, it's up to the courts. The cops were just doing their jobs.

Assuming they don't need to go to the hospital first, next stop for arrestees after the squad car was booking at CJC. Here, jail staff carried out the usual chores like photographs, fingerprinting, explanation of charges and the like. A body scan like at the airport was part of the entry process.

The scanner at CJC came courtesy of funding from the U.S Immigration and Customs Enforcement (ICE). At over $200,000 a pop these machines aren't for Mayberry's jail.

The scanner largely replaced the need for strip searches. Considering the hygienic state of many of my patients, everybody was in favor of that. The seven-second scan shoots a 1 mm thick beam of low dose x-rays through the miscreant, while an automated moving platform shuttles him through. Compared to the fifteen minutes that an ordinary strip search takes, this is a huge help. It helped the person being scanned too. He could keep all his clothes on except his shoes.

The deputies liked it because they didn't have to touch the offender before the scan. This protected them from getting punctured from hidden needles, razor blades and the like.

Some were worried about the radiation exposure, but the dose from the scanner was 1/400th of what you get in a routine chest x-ray. If that's not low enough, one scan compared to about 1/25th the radiation dose that all of us get every day just by hanging around on planet Earth.

Edna Banks was intoxicated when she drove her 2002 Toyota Camry over a fire hydrant and clipped the edge of a 7-11 before wiping out a

Goodwill collection box. Not being too clear on what to do next, she was arrested while gathering up old clothes and shoes and piling them on the crushed donation station. Maybe nobody would notice.

Edna arrived for booking at CJC in an outraged snit flanked by a pair of deputies.

"Get your hands off me you jackasses!" Edna squirmed and jerked against the restraining arms. "Turn me loose! I'm a lady, dammit. I'm a fucking lady!"

After the initial questioning Edna was loaded into the scanner. Something opaque showed between her breasts. She was questioned again.

"It's just my damn bra, you idiots," she explained. Unwilling to take her word for this, a female deputy searched for and removed a sizable packet of cocaine from Edna's undergarment. An easy score for the scanner.

Besides obvious items like weapons, the scanner was good at picking out hidden illegal drugs in body cavities. Balloons, often made of condoms or the fingers of latex gloves, were filled with cocaine or heroin and swallowed either to transport them or in panic when arrest was imminent.

The balloons routinely turned up in stomachs, vaginas or rectums. On an abdominal x-ray hashish looks dark, while cocaine is about the same density as stool. Heroin looks like air. Here's a tip: balloons filled with drugs dissolved in water are damned hard to see without special scanners.

Jimmie Merced presented an interesting case when he was scanned. A large balloon showed up in his abdomen, but he insisted that he'd swallowed nothing. He was brought to medical for me to examine him. He plunked himself on the exam table with a distinctly shifty look.

"Mr. Merced, can I take a look at your belly?"

After some hemming and hawing, he lifted his shirt. He had a colostomy.

I looked at it. I looked at him. "Jimmie?" I said.

He screwed up his mouth and stared back.

"Should we have a peek?"

"I got a colostomy."

"Got that," I said, pointing to the colostomy bag. "Let's see what's behind door number one."

With the encouragement of the two deputies, Jimmie relented and removed the bag. "See?" he said, "Nothin'."

"Let's clean things up a bit and have a look inside."

"Inside? You ain't touchin' me inside."

I held my palms up. "Your choice. You want a glove?"

He snorted and stuck his fingers in the opening, extracting a latex balloon filled with a powder.

"Happy?" he said.

"Ecstatic."

Balloons like these presented a real problem because if one broke, the prisoner could receive a lethal dose of the narcotic. Sending him or her to the hospital for surgical removal risked the same thing. Intestinal obstruction was a companion problem. Usually the prisoner was placed in a "dry cell," a cell with no toilet or running water, and we waited for nature to take its course. The deputies drew straws for who got to search for the balloons.

Not everyone gets picked up in intake, and some offenders would rather roll the dice than admit to a drug charge. Not long ago an offender was found dead in his cell. The autopsy revealed a level of heroin 8,000 times the lethal dose.

Verla Saiz was booked into CJC one July evening on a vagrancy charge and assigned to one of the women's housing units. At morning rounds she was slow to respond to the call for count. As the day progressed she became less and less responsive. The deputies brought her down to medical.

Verla could barely sit on my exam table. Her blood pressure was low, her breathing shallow. A quick neurologic exam showed pinpoint pupils, and her speech, barely audible, was slurred. Off to the hospital.

In the process of inserting a Foley urinary catheter, the ER doctors found bags of narcotics in her vagina, one of which was leaking. A close call.

The nurse midwife poked her head around the corner. "Doc, could you come in here a minute?"

Usually the midwife does her own thing, but today she needed a witness. She introduced Lori Cordell, who was draped in a compromising position on her exam table. "Ms. Cordell has been complaining about a persistent vaginal discharge." This didn't seem to be in my line, but I stayed silent and attentive.

The midwife held up a plastic bag of white powder, which later proved to be methamphetamine. I eye rolled toward Ms. Cordell's posterior and raised my eyebrows inquiringly. The midwife nodded.

"I think we've found the cause of your infection," I said.

Ms. Cordell raised her head and saw the packet. "Oh, I completely forgot that was there!" she exclaimed. And I'm sure she was telling the truth.

Along the same lines, many staff wouldn't sit near the chairs in intake on "hooker night." I haven't checked it out personally, but apparently they got pretty sticky. I considered myself warned.

Assuming no medical catastrophes or last-minute attempts at flight while being booked, the prisoners advanced to the intake nurse. The nurse noted any health issues and set appointments for chronic care clinics or for more immediate health care.

The nurse put the prisoner's medications into the EMR system or forwarded any unusual or questionable items to me or the nurse practitioner. She noted anything about pregnancy, communicable diseases, or present drug and alcohol use. We didn't routinely test for drugs at intake, so sometimes there was a surprise a day or two later when they went into withdrawal. Actually it's not much of a surprise, just something we looked out for on everyone.

Getting arrested is a stressful process, so it was common for patients to register high blood pressures in intake. When the sheets from these patients crossed my desk, I gave them a few days to cool down and get a couple more readings before I set up an appointment to manage the problem.

Stress showed up in other ways too. We had more than one baby delivered in intake.

Since felons often used aliases, the nurses confirmed as best they could the actual name(s) of new prisoners. We got plenty of nicknames like Monster, Cowboy, Tweety, DaDa, Jenga, and Suspect. Some were more off-the-wall like Dr. ZLove (a lover of zombies?), Shortshot (an apparent reference to genital anatomy), Pitstop (a frequent visitor to the bathroom) or Bobblehead (use your imagination).

My favorite was the girl named Shithead. She said it was pronounced she-the-add, but looking at the booking sheet, I think I had it right the first time.

NINE

BONDO

You can't bail yourself out of prison, but jail is another matter. A new inmate arrives at the jail due to "probable cause." In other words, the police think he's committed some kind of crime. No matter what he was arrested for, it's the prosecutor who decides what the charges are and even if the matter will be carried on to court.

If the crime isn't too serious, he may be allowed to post bail immediately and walk. Otherwise he may have to wait a day or two for a bail hearing, where a judge can decide whether to set bail or not.

There weren't any hard-and-fast rules about setting the amount of bail, but there were guidelines. It might be $25,000 for perjury, $100,000 for manslaughter, and $1,000,000 for kidnapping. It's designed to assure the person's appearance for a court date where guilt or innocence can be determined.

The type of offense was only one parameter in determining bail. The judge also looked at the defendant's criminal record, his history of showing up for prior court appearances, whether he had ties in the community, and whether he was a danger to himself or others.

Bail could take different forms. The simplest was a cash bail where the accused paid the full amount of the bail himself. Some courts even took checks and credit cards.

If the accused didn't have the cash on hand, he could get a surety bond. In this case he usually got a friend or relative to contact a bail agent, also known as a bail bondsman. In exchange for some collateral like real estate or personal property, the bondsman would arrange to put up the bail amount. He charged a 10 percent premium for this service.

The bondsman was backed by a special insurance company that pledged to pay the amount of the bond if the accused didn't appear for his court date (about 20 percent don't). If that happens, the bondsman was out the money and was unhappy. He might employ a bounty hunter, or bail enforcement agent, as they preferred to be called. If the bounty hunter successfully tracked down the no-show, he typically collected 10 to 20 percent of the bail bond amount.

Bounty hunters can make pretty good money, upwards of $80,000 per year if they work hard, but the work isn't pleasant. Still, they're often more effective than the police, nabbing about 90 percent of their quarries.

To be fair, bounty hunters have advantages the police don't enjoy. When an accused person signs the bail bond agreement, he signs away some constitutional rights. He agrees that he can be arrested by the bail bond agent anywhere at any time. Bounty hunters don't need to worry about Miranda rights or getting a search warrant. All they have to do to enter the fugitive's home is to be sure the fugitive lives there. They don't need to worry about jurisdiction, except they can't go outside the United States.

Although not an office job, the danger inherent in chasing criminals doesn't usually loom large for the bounty hunters. The people they're chasing aren't violent criminals or they wouldn't have made bail in the first place. Also, only a small percentage resists arrest when they're caught and then only by trying to escape again.

For minor offenses the arresting officer may not book the accused at all, but will write a citation telling him to appear in court on a certain date. The big advantage here is avoiding all the time and paperwork of a formal booking. Obviously this is only for minor offenses.

At the bail hearing, the judge may release the accused on his own recognizance. This means the accused doesn't have to come up with any money to make bail. He does have to make a really good impression on the judge though.

In 1988 Colorado made domestic violence (DV) a status crime. What this means is DV isn't a crime in itself, but a label that's tacked on to whatever else the person is arrested for. A status crime means you have to go to jail for DV until you appear before a judge, who explains your charges to you and decides whether to allow any bond or not.

This came about after a man accused of DV made a bond of $20,000 but was allowed to leave jail. He went right home, raped his wife in numerous inventive ways and bludgeoned her to death with a telephone receiver. After that, anyone arrested for DV spent time in jail.

Another type of bail is a property bond. Here, the accused puts up property to secure the bail instead of cash. The court takes a lien on the property and can foreclose to collect the bail if the accused doesn't show.

Just like in the movies, you get a free call at booking. If whoever you're calling isn't available, they'll give you another one, within reason. These calls aren't monitored, but the ones made from the housing pods are.

Before you can make calls in jail, you need to fill out an "approved call list." These are five people who are vetted by the police before you're allowed to call them. If someone on your list isn't approved for one reason or another, you can pick someone else up to the limit of five. Better make one of them your lawyer.

Now the jail staff will classify you. This means they try to put you in a housing pod with people in criminal classes similar to yours. Petty criminals one way, violent ones another, crazies to a third. They also look at any history of prior escapes, misbehavior in previous incarcerations, criminal history and such.

At CJC each housing pod has a gestalt. Alpha 1 and 3 receive the bad-ass females, while their male counterparts get Charlie and Delta pods. Females with lesser offenses get Echo 2 and the men go to the tower. Mental health claims Alpha 2 for females and Bravo 2 for males. The idea is not only to separate males and females, but also the different levels of offender, keeping the hard cases away from the newbies.

So you don't get mixed up, everyone gets color-coded scrubs to wear: orange for felonies, blue for misdemeanors, red for juveniles, teal for mental health, green for trustees, and white for kitchen workers. Turtle suits are a special kind of wardrobe. These are heavily quilted ponchos worn by patients who have threatened to harm themselves or are otherwise deranged.

Footwear is easy. Everyone gets orange sandals. There is an exception for diabetics. They can get a kind of cheap blue slip-on with an arch support like a pool table. Although the sandals are really more comfortable, everyone seems to want the blue jobs since they aren't "standard issue." Anything for status.

TEN

THE CAFETERIA

Territorial prison in Cañon City has a culinary training program that services a small cafeteria open to staff for breakfast and lunch. With a nod to the ethnicity of many of the inmates, the menu features Mexican items in addition to the usual grill offerings.

No other Colorado prison has such a facility, so I was overjoyed to see a mini-cafeteria right next to medical at CJC. Maybe I wouldn't have to brown bag it every day with my frozen Lean Cuisine offerings.

The cafeteria was a spacious room with a mural of a Parisian street scene occupying one wall. I could find deputies at break sitting at the tables scattered around the room next to the free coffee and soda dispensers. All we needed was donuts.

The serving line opened at about 11 a.m. with a special of the day prepared by inmate chefs. Typical fare consisted of baked chicken, ziti, or mystery meat with overcooked vegetables on the side. Popular days featured pizza or corn dogs, a favorite of Wendy, my HSA. Although the inmates tried their best, we're dealing with prison food bought with state money in bulk. Wolfgang Puck has nothing to worry about.

Most of the time I stuck with my frozen delicacies, not only because of the food quality but also because I frequently got hit up for free medical opinions. It's the prison equivalent of getting buttonholed at a cocktail party. Michael, a diabetic awaiting trial on drug charges, was a case in point.

"Hey, Doc. My sugars are running high in the afternoon. Think we could bump the insulin a little in the morning?"

"Sound like we might have to. When's your next appointment?"

"Next week, but I thought maybe you could just fix it now."

"There's no computer here in the cafeteria."

"Well, no, I mean when you get back to the clinic. Just take a minute."

"Okay, I'll look at it. Maybe I could get lunch first?"

Now if I blew Michael off I could probably count on getting the burned piece of whatever was being served. Worse, I might end up on the revenge list with certain unmentionable contaminants added to my food in the future. It happens.

Sometimes the requests for instant consults were useful. Aaron was serving six months for car theft.

"Hi, Aaron. What's good today?"

"Hey, Doc. Special is baked lasagna."

"Your recipe?"

"You bet. Made it myself. Hey, you know I been having diarrhea something fierce. Think you could get me something for that?"

(replacing the tray) "Diarrhea, eh? Maybe I should see you over in the clinic for that. Drop me a kite."

"Okay, Doc. Want some of this?"

"Dieting, Aaron, thanks just the same. Think I'll just get a glass of water."

The cafeteria was reserved for staff only. Inmates were out of luck except working the serving line and cadging whatever they can back in the kitchen. It's one of the hardships of jail life that the food, without exception, is terrible.

Food for the prisoners at CJC is the worst I've encountered in my nine years working in corrections. Granted, none of the prisons is going to win any Michelin awards, but CJC seems to have reached a culinary nadir. In 2005 a group of inmates filed a lawsuit over "spoiled milk, rotten fruit, and watered-down soup that tastes like dishwater." You can guess how far that court action got.

The cafeteria might rate a D+ in industrial food service, but the trays that made the rounds of the housing pods weren't even that good. Two slices of white bread, a lump of mystery meat, an orange and a carton of orange drink was lunch pretty much every day. I'd tell you about dinner, but I never could identify the ingredients. Just try to control a diabetic with a solid carbohydrate diet. Somebody was making money off this food delivery. Just sayin'...

ELEVEN

THE FLOOD

I dashed through the employee entrance on a blustery, rainy Colorado morning, shedding my raincoat and draping it over a gooseneck lamp in my office. Sitting down at the computer I started to log in, when I noticed a splashing sound under the desk.

I thought at first that Stacy had spilled her Big Gulp, but no, I heard dripping. I peered under the desk, finding a huge puddle around the computer and water pouring in a steady stream from above. The stream emanated from a watermelon-sized bubble at the top of the sheetrock wall. *This can't be good.*

I realized that, even worse, I was sitting in a pool of water creeping up the side of a large electric appliance. I pulled the plug on the computer and stepped back from the aquatic Sword of Damocles.

Although the inmate tower is relatively new, the administrative portion of CJC is not. The aging flat roof had burst a seam right over my desk and it was still raining like hell outside.

We called the maintenance guys while watching the balloon slowly dissect along the top of the wall. Feeling pretty good about handling the emergency without electrocution or drowning, Wendy, Denise and I waited for the cavalry.

Wendy said, "What's on the other side of this wall?" Hmm, hadn't thought of that. So we walked around and found a storeroom that shared my wall. This contained all the supplies for the clinic. Damage from a drenching here would have approached six figures, so my office was forgotten while we formed a human chain to empty out the room.

Fortunately, I guess, the balloon burst in my office first and the storeroom was saved. The maintenance guys said the needed repairs were beyond their pay grade. We'd have to have a roofing company put on a new one. Can you guess how that turned out?

The sheriff's office decided that since Colorado was having a drought anyway, there was really no reason to put all that money into a new roof. Six months later I was still stuck with wallpaper that looked like elephant skin. When it rained I made sure to wear my rubber shoes.

TWELVE

DETOX

Hospitals hate drunks and addicts. They consume loads of medical resources in emergency rooms, and they come back again and again. Many have other significant medical problems because of their lifestyle and most are broke.

As a humanitarian (read: cost-saving) measure, the local hospitals got together to fund a detox facility where they could direct (read: dump) these individuals. The goal of detoxification is to manage acute intoxications and withdrawal involving drugs or alcohol. Ideally you want to motivate the patient to enter treatment.

The detox center was located on the grounds of the CJC. As such, the sheriff was sort of responsible for administration. I say *sort of* because the detox patients weren't arrested and couldn't be treated as criminals. As the medical director at CJC, I became the detox specialist by default.

There are a couple of types of detox facilities. What you would think of as a real live detox facility is called a medical model. In this model the facility is staffed by detox specialists with medical training, along with physician supervision. They treat impaired individuals in settings ranging from hospitals to free-standing clinics and dispense medication to assist in withdrawal. We don't have one of these.

What we have is called a social model. It's a kind of glorified drunk tank. The detox facility can't dispense prescription drugs from its own pharmacy because we can't have a pharmacy. We don't have a license. To get a license, we'd have to (gasp) spend money, and that just wasn't going to happen.

To be fair, the license is expensive, and we'd have to upgrade the personnel staffing the clinic. Instead of physicians and RNs, we had LPNs and nurse's aides. Without a pharmacy and personnel to administer medications, we were reduced to hand-holding and a few over-the-counter drugs.

People around Colorado Springs who had overindulged were brought to the detox center by ambulance or the cops. We'd get their history (although we knew most of them pretty well), do a physical assessment of their degree of intoxication, and put them to bed. Welcome home.

The detox center occupied a dumbbell-shaped prefab hut on a concrete slab next to the main CJC building. One side for the men and the other for the women with staff sandwiched in between. Each housing unit consisted of a nurse's station and a large open area filled with rows of beds.

If people were actually arrested while intoxicated, we'd have them over in a medical cell at CJC. Otherwise they'd come in to detox, sleep it off, and leave in a day or two.

A few came via court order to be involuntarily committed. These IC candidates came with letters from their family or significant others detailing what they'd been up to for the past several years in a downward spiral with drugs or alcohol.

The next stop for an IC was an interview with me to see if I agreed that they needed to be committed for the good of themselves and others. It was a sad exercise. I didn't see a single person who had insight into what the addition had done and was doing to them and the people around them.

I'd hear all kinds of excuses from "I've got it under control now," to "I'll get into a program next week," to "They just don't understand what I'm going through." They all said they had their addiction under control now after failing in programs the last five or six times. They all looked forward to being in a program to get rid of the addiction…next week.

The stories I got were beyond horrendous. The letters I read were usually from mothers or fathers detailing years of out-of-control drug and alcohol use with suicide attempts, car crashes, assaults, sexual abuse, and theft. If you saw one of these stories on television, you'd turn it off as being totally unbelievable.

Laura Hartnett was a 23-year-old woman admitted to the detox unit for an IC evaluation. I read through a two-page statement by her parents pleading for her commitment into a rehab program. These statements are in "just the facts, ma'am" format, but it was painfully clear the torture that these people had endured trying to salvage their daughter. Scrapes with juvenile authorities over alcohol and marijuana dotted her mid-teen years. In high school she was in trouble with cocaine, both buying and selling. She clashed with her parents over promiscuous sex and wrecked a stolen car when she was seventeen. At eighteen she moved out to live with her 29-year-old lover, who pimped her out for favors and drugs. Heroin became the focus of her life.

Laura burglarized her parents' house on several occasions to gain items to pawn. By age twenty-one she'd attempted suicide twice. Her parents paid for admission to private addiction treatment facilities on three occasions, but she'd left each one after only a few days.

Now she sat across from me in a tiny conference room, barely adequate to hold a desk and two chairs. Auburn hair brushed back and body recently scrubbed, Laura sat straight in the chair with her knees and palms pressed tightly together in a bunch, as if she was keeping her legs from jumping. Though an attractive young woman, her brown eyes radiated a tense anxiety.

I took my seat and extended a hand. "Miss Hartnett, I'm Doctor Wright." She pried a hand loose from clutching her knee and shot it out.

"I'm so glad to see you, Doctor Wright. I feel so much better now."

"How so?"

She leaned forward earnestly. "I know I've had some problems in the past, but I think I've finally got a handle on them. I guess I wasn't ready to hear what people were saying before, but now I know I'll be okay."

"You've had some problems with drugs..."

She fanned her hand in front of her face, waving off the question. "I know. It was so stupid. I see how destructive it was. I'm never going to do anything like that again."

"Getting drugs out of your life can be tough. Do you think getting some help with that would be a good idea?"

"Oh, I've seen the counselors, and I think they're absolutely right. I'm planning to go back to one of the programs next week, just to touch base. They've really helped a lot."

"Are you thinking about hurting yourself?"

"Oh, no. I would never do something like that."

"You were in the emergency room a month ago with an overdose."

"That was just a mistake. I was just sitting around with some friends, and we were celebrating a guy's birthday. I think maybe somebody spiked my drink."

"What do you think about getting into a program now?"

Laura looked at me as if I'd just asked her if she'd like to sleep in a roomful of rattlesnakes. "Oh, no. I don't need that. I mean I appreciate your concern, but I'm done with that stuff. I'm clean, and I know I can make it this time, and I've got some really great friends to help out if I need them."

"These the same ones who spiked your drink?"

"Not those losers. I've got some good friends that have been through rehab and know all that stuff."

You can see how this is going. Laura will tell me anything to keep from being involuntarily committed into a month-long rehab program. It's typical that these patients will admit to previous transgressions. After all, I'm sitting there with the records right in front of me. They'll also state unequivocally that they've seen the light and are miraculously cured of a decade of drug abuse, assault, theft, and self-destruction.

I filled out the papers that went to the judge to determine if Laura should be involuntarily committed for treatment. I can't imagine that any I saw were turned loose, but that part was out of my hands. Theoretically I could be called to court to give testimony in a commitment case, but it never happened.

People being held like this weren't free to leave like the rest of the detox patients. One skinny young man almost made his escape by squeezing through a junction between two walls into a utility room, climbing up and over inside an air duct and ending up stuck above the furnace. Good thing it was summer.

Apparently the undersheriff, Paula Presley, had some deep connections to the detox clients. I arrived at work one morning to an urgent message from the charge nurse.

"Presley says she wants you to do an IC evaluation right away. The papers have to be in by noon."

"Okay," I said. "I'll go over right now. You know where to find me."

I segued over to the detox unit to see the young lady, a Miss Elbers, but nobody knew anything about her or the IC evaluation. No papers. Nada. I checked my watch. Nine o'clock.

"We've got some time," I said. "I'll get clinic started, and you call me as soon as you find the paperwork."

Nine turned into ten with no word. I called detox. "Did you find the papers on Miss Elbers?" I asked. Yes, they had. I thought to ask why they hadn't called me, but instead just put the clinic on hold and traveled back to the unit.

No sooner had I set foot in detox than I got a stat page from the medical unit with a cardiac emergency. Back I went, feeling a little like a yo-yo.

As these things sometimes happen, I had not one but two cardiac emergencies. There were streamers of EKG paper and forests of crash carts and IV bags littering the clinic. In the midst of the chaos, an aide came in with a message from the undersheriff.

"Presley wants to know why the IC evaluation isn't done yet," she said.

I couldn't believe it. "I guess it's because I'm up to my armpits in alligators at the moment. Tell her that cardiac emergencies trump IC evaluations. I'll get it done as soon as I can."

Once the smoke cleared, I returned to the detox unit and did the evaluation. Eleven-fifteen. Papers filed. Deadline met. Crisis averted.

Presley didn't think so. She said that I should have done the IC evaluation that she wanted first and then taken care of whatever pesky medical problems

I had later. I was stupefied. What can you say to someone who thinks filling out her paperwork is more important than a heart attack (or two)?

They say that Steve Jobs radiated a reality-distortion field that could bend facts to fit his perception of the way things ought to be. I think Presley could give him a run for his money.

We had lots of frequent fliers in detox. Over 500 patients passed through every month. Every time a patient was admitted to the facility, the nurses filled out papers about their history and condition. The accumulated charts of many patients ran to four or five volumes. It wasn't unusual at all for a patient to drink all day, come to detox to sleep it off overnight, and leave in the morning to start the cycle all over again.

I got to know some of the patients from signing off on their charts. I was signing the nightly visits of Jurryt Palmiro and noticed he hadn't been in for a week. I remembered him because of the odd first name.

"Did we cure Mr. Palmiro?' I asked one of the nurses, indicating the chart.

"He died last week," she said. "They found him frozen down in Memorial Park."

The detox staff did the best they could, but they're emptying the ocean with a teacup. Most of their addicted patients thought everything was okay, despite all evidence to the contrary. Denial, rationalization, fatalism, self-destructive tendencies, and poverty all played a part in keeping the addicts addicted. I'd like to say "And the solution is…," but I don't have any.

Thirteen

The Secret of Cell One

The cells in medical were numbered 1 through 16. Cell 1 was immediately across from the nurses' station and was reserved for the patients most in need of close observation. Unfortunately these were often the most disruptive patients.

Drunks, addicts in withdrawal, and crazies all came to Cell 1 at least until they were judged to be free of acute medical problems. These were the people who yell, scream, pound the door, urinate and defecate on the floor and walls and generally serve as pains in the ass for everyone within earshot. Including me.

My exam room/office sat about twenty yards from Cell 1, so I got to participate in hearing all their ranting, pounding and screaming. In the movies this is where the mental health practitioners troop in and fill the bozo with psychotropic drugs. Not here.

"It's behavioral," my mental health colleagues would say. "It's not a mental illness."

"It's creating mental illness for everyone around them," I'd respond. "Can't you just give him something to pacify him a little? I can't hear myself think."

"Nope. Wish we could help. Call us if he gets psychotic." Then they'd retire to their warren behind two locked doors in another—quiet—part of the clinic. Thanks, guys.

I do appreciate that the MH folks can't just go injecting people willy-nilly, but the Cell 1 residents would be first on my list if they could. I admired the ability of the nurses at their station to keep functioning in the midst of the bedlam. They had to endure the patient slamming his face up against the window of the cell, making living Halloween masks and exhibiting his endowments.

The only time we could really intervene was if the occupant was in danger of hurting himself. Even then the security staff was severely limited in what they could do. They could only use restraints for a short period of time, maybe a couple of hours at most. The patient, if restrained, had to have a full set of checks every fifteen minutes to make sure he wasn't strangling himself. It just wasn't worth it.

One of the nurses showed me the "loose brick" trick in one of these situations. She'd tell the patient confidentially that Cell 1 held a secret. There was a loose brick in the wall somewhere that led to the outside and warned him not to take it out. Stupid as it sounds, many of them bought it and spent hours in blessed silence probing each cinder block in the cell for the loose one that led to freedom.

Considering the occupants, Cell 1 could get pretty nasty. The cell doesn't have any fixtures like a sink or toilet, just a drain in the middle of the floor. Hosing down the room is a regular necessity, otherwise your shoes tend to stick to the floor from whatever bodily fluids coat it. It's gross. Sorry I mentioned it.

Cell 1 also has secret healing powers. For some reason, sudden paralysis from the waist down is a popular malady in the jail. Jay Noonan, arrested for domestic violence, was a recent case.

Jay rolled into the clinic in a wheelchair, flanked by two deputies. We maneuvered him into my office and we talked.

"I understand your legs are paralyzed, Mr. Noonan. How did that get started?"

"I dunno, Doc, Just woke up like this."

"No kidding? You seem pretty put together for a guy who woke up paralyzed."

"Yeah, well, I mean I'm upset, of course."

"Of course. I guess you're peeing on yourself too. Crapped your pants?"

"Oh, no. Nothin' like that. Just the legs."

Pulling out a wicked-looking needle, I smile. "Probably can't feel anything down there either."

Jay's eyes widened. "Oh, no. I can feel everything just fine."

"Let's check this out." I do a physical exam and check reflexes and such. "Looks pretty good."

"I can't work like this, Doc." Ah, the light dawns.

"Probably not, but I've seen cases similar to this that got better pretty quickly. We'll get the treatment started today."

"Anything, Doc. I'm really messed up."

The treatment consists on putting Jay on a mattress in Cell 1 and leaving him alone. Pretty soon, he'll need to pee. Staying in character, Jay drags himself agonizingly over to the drain hole and relieves himself. Not used to this much physical exertion, he now has to drag himself back.

Jay's getting hungry. Part of this advanced therapy is placing his meal tray on the opposite side of the cell. Again with the dragging, although he's beginning to use his knees in a surreptitious crawl.

Reality is setting in after a few hours of neglect. Jay realizes the gambit isn't working and <MIRACLE> Jay stands up and walks to the door, demanding to go back to the housing pod so he won't miss his basketball game. The mystical healing powers of Cell 1 manifest once more.

Cell 1 worked for all kinds of bogus ailments. Seizures, horrible excruciating total body pain, attacks of cancer, and the general feel-bads all succumbed to the magic of benign neglect. Once I was convinced that the patient's complaint was bullshit, transfer to the therapeutic effects of Cell 1 moved to the top of the list.

Offenders had strategies to outfox Cell 1. We had one who would sit quietly in the cell until he'd had enough. Then he's rush to the door, pounding and shouting, "Fire! Fire!" A little unnerving at first, but like *The Boy Who Cried Wolf*, it only worked once.

The nurses had their strategies too. When an offender was raucous, a nurse would tiptoe to the door, tap lightly and, holding a finger to her lips, whisper, "Shhh. You'll wake the baby." It's amazing how often it worked.

Darren Brown was a "behavior problem." He liked to stick things up his penis. I never found out what his original crime was, but his hobby took center stage.

Darren was inventive. After exhausting the objects more readily at hand like beads, pencil erasers and pebbles, he started in with wadded bits of paper and folded sections of plastic coffee cup lids.

I would expect it to hurt like hell, but Darren apparently loved it. My mental health colleagues informed me that it was an auto-erotic act, but I think Darren just liked the effect on everyone else.

If I could extract the foreign body I would, but often he'd gotten things piled in there so deeply that we'd have to send him to the ER for the urologist to remove them.

We put Darren in Cell 1 for observation and so we could take everything away that he could conceivably use. Darren was smarter than we were. He unraveled threads and small strips of cloth from his blanket, rolled them up and used them. He managed to extract flakes of cinder block from the walls. He used his own hair.

Mental health said that his actions weren't a mental illness, but rather a behavior to control the rest of us. And he liked it. Translation: We're not getting involved with this yahoo.

Cell 1 didn't work on Darren. It just made him more inventive. We finally shunted him off to a prison facility, and good riddance.

FOURTEEN

THE REVENGE OF THE BUNKS

I never really appreciated how dangerous beds could be until I started to work in prisons. Not a week goes by that someone doesn't come to medical with bruises and lacerations from falling out of bed. Even people on lower bunks come in with bloody noses, black eyes, concussions and even broken bones.

Second only to falling out of bed are those who fall on the stairs or slip in the bathroom, sustaining similar injuries. It's pretty amazing. You'd almost think someone had beaten them up.

I had one patient who came to medical with a forehead laceration and bruises on his chest. He told me he fell out of bed. In the middle of the day. We returned him to the housing pod, and would you believe he slipped getting into his bunk and got a laceration above the other eye. Talk about bad luck.

Admonishing him to be careful, we again sent him back to the housing pod. He at least lasted until the next day, when he came down with a broken jaw. Fell taking a shower and hit his face on a faucet. This got him a trip to the oral surgeon. He got his jaws wired shut, which probably helped in preventing further injuries. In jail, as in life, it's often better to keep your mouth shut.

If a patient had a fight, we could put him in protective custody or at least change his housing pod. Since we dealt with skewed personalities to begin with, patients took their attitudes along with them when changing pods. It often meant that accidents just happened in a different location.

Jails aren't pleasant places to begin with. Add overcrowding in a population already dripping with testosterone, and you're going to have some disagreements. Things usually got rolling for medical when someone called a Code Blue.

Code Blue meant everyone RAN to where the action is. You could literally get run down by puffing deputies if you were negligent enough to stand in a hallway. Best to just peek out a doorway.

Fights, man down, or medical emergencies brought a swift cadre of deputies and medical personnel to deal with the crisis. Being old and slow, I usually waited for the situation to stabilize until I ambled in.

If a Code Blue occurred in the tower, things were a little different. The tower had three levels with four flights of stairs per level. If we got the call from one of the upper floors, the nursing staff took the elevator.

Most Code Blues turned out to be minor incidents or false alarms. If not, in about ten minutes I'd see a couple of roughed-up inmates escorted through medical to separate holding cells. I repaired any damage from the altercation, and after the sutures and bandages the miscreants got some time out to contemplate the error of their ways.

Other Code Blues were more serious. Seizures were pretty common, chest pain less so. Most of the time I waited in medical for the troops to bring their trophies back for examination, but sometimes I made house calls.

Terrance Lewis was back in jail for the third time that year for burglary. He didn't want to be there and let everyone know it. Finally he felt a demonstration was in order, and he took a dive headfirst off the second-level tier in his housing unit. He did a good job, and I was called up to the unit.

Terrance was lying unconscious in a pool of blood. Head lacerations always bleed like hell anyway, but this looked worse. His head was actually misshapen from contact with the concrete floor. I checked his neurologic signs and wasn't encouraged. We got him strapped to a back board with his head and neck stabilized, and sent him off to the hospital.

I really didn't expect him to be back, but about ten days later he showed up on my clinic roster. He still had a hell of a headache and walked unsteadily, but against all odds he was alive. Truly amazing.

What appeared to be a lethal plunge could turn out to be relatively minor. Another prisoner who dove headfirst to the ground from the second tier only ended up knocking his front teeth out.

A young female car thief named Angela Brodkins tried the same thing. Sort of. The deputies were putting Angela in her cell on the second tier when she just disappeared. They scrambled to the rail and saw Angela contorted on the concrete below. Code Blue.

I examined Angela, but she was in excruciating pain, writhing and screaming. Ah well, off to the ER for evaluation of her injuries. Turns out there weren't any. Wow, that was lucky. Maybe Angela bounced.

A review of the videos showed the deputies turning away to unlock the cell. Angela, quick like a bunny, hopped over the rail and lowered herself to the first tier. She lay down and arranged herself on the floor awaiting discovery. I'm not sure what point she was trying to make, but she did get a free trip to the hospital and some nice pain meds courtesy of the ER staff.

We had our share of persons trying to harm themselves. One prisoner managed to get a staple and scraped away at his arm in secret until he actually hit an artery. The cell looked like it was spray-painted by a maniac—and I guess it was. The nurses that had to enter the cell ended up bagging their clothes and wearing leftover scrubs from the inmates the rest of the day.

Jails are mostly for holding accused persons prior to their trials. There were lots of people there for short-term sentences as well, a month or so. The jail just isn't set up for long-term confinement. The average stay is just shy of a month, but occasionally we had longer stays.

Mary Cummins was an obese diabetic woman with chronic lung disease from years of smoking. She had three or four other major illnesses, but her most distinguishing feature was her narcissism. The world revolved around Mary.

She was in jail for wrapping her daughter's infant girl in duct tape and placing her in the bathtub under a cold shower until the child was nearly dead of hypothermia. The infant's crime? She had knocked Mary's glass of Jack Daniels over while crawling on the floor.

The child had permanent brain damage and will be institutionalized for the rest of her life. Her mother, Mary's daughter, didn't intervene during this water boarding because she didn't want to upset her mother.

Mary was convicted and sentenced to forty years in prison, but for an unknown reason she was to spend the first two years incarcerated at CJC. I try not to be judgmental with my patients, but Mary was an exception. If Jabba the Hutt landed in CJC, he could be Mary's twin.

Because of her numerous ailments she had to be housed in medical with her own private cell. She played everything to the hilt, demanding special diets and referrals to specialists for her real and imagined medical demands. Constantly whining and complaining about everything, I couldn't help gnashing my teeth thinking of the little girl she'd tortured and robbed of a life.

Mary had a lot in common with my old patients at Colorado State Penitentiary (CSP), the state's maximum-security prison. One constant shared by nearly all the CSP inmates was a complete lack of empathy. They had no feeling whatsoever for the people they had injured with their crimes.

If they shot someone while attempting to steal his car, it was the victim's fault for not immediately giving them what they wanted. "He made me shoot him because he wouldn't give me the keys," would be a typical comment. Mary was the same way. It was clear that she gave her granddaughter no more thought than she might a petty annoyance. I came close to hating Mary, and it took all my professional willpower to tend to her medical needs without some thought of retaliation. The words of my first warden at CSP came back to me: "People go to prison *as* punishment, not *for* punishment." It wasn't my place to punish Mary; I was her doctor.

Mary was a demanding narcissist. No medical care was ever good enough for her. She treated the infirmary like her private hotel and the nurses as personal servants. I'll admit that most of her niggling demands fell on my deaf ears when I thought of the little girl she'd brutalized. I like to work with my patients to make their lives as healthful and comfortable as you can be in confinement, but in Mary's case I just didn't care. For one of the few times in my life, I wouldn't have been upset to come in and find her dead in her cell.

That I could feel this way about a patient bothered me. It went against all my training, but I had to recognize that the emotion was real. I remembered a *grook*, a short poem, by the Danish writer, Piet Hein, which seemed to cover the situation:

An Ethical Grook

I see
and I hear
and I speak no evil;
I carry
no malice
within my breast;
yet quite without
wishing
a man to the Devil
one may be
permitted
to hope for the best.

Fifteen

Packing Heat

Roger, one of the deputies, lounged in my door while waiting to take some prisoners back to the floor. "Say, what kinda gun you got, Doc?"

I looked up from my typing. "None. Well, I've got a .357, but I haven't shot it in years. I don't think there's any ammunition for it anyway."

"You're kidding, right? Working with these guys, you should have a gun."

I thought back to Ralphie in *A Christmas Story*. "Probably put my eye out, Roger."

"No, really, Doc. You remember that guy that shot the head of DOC?"

I did remember the guy who shot and killed Tom Clements, the executive director of Colorado Department of Corrections. Evan Ebel was one of my patients at CSP, the Colorado supermax. He had been released four years early due to a clerical mistake and had assassinated Clements when he answered his door in March of 2013.

Ebel, a member of the white supremacist 211 Crew gang, killed another man and wounded a sheriff's deputy before being killed himself in a shootout with lawmen in Texas. The judge in a trial of his accomplice who purchased the gun for him described Ebel as an intelligent sociopath, and I expect that's about right. I wasn't that impressed with his intelligence when I saw him as a patient, but he wasn't trying to charm me then.

"Yeah, Roger, I remember him. You think somebody's coming after me?"

"Just sayin', Doc. Better prepared."

Well, maybe he was right. Denise, my director of nursing, told me she was going to get a concealed weapon permit. I asked her about it.

"You need to take a course first," she said. "There's one in two weeks that I'm taking. Why don't you come?"

Well, why not? I signed up.

Two weeks later Denise and I met a half dozen other potential Dirty Harrys at a private shooting range outside Colorado Springs. It was winter and the classroom, a plywood shack, had not been assembled with great care. Wind whistled through the cracks where the walls didn't quite join and an inadequate kerosene heater gave only illusory comfort.

The instructor knew his gun law, that's for sure. We spent the better part of the day learning all the regulations about when we could shoot people. After a late lunch in the car with the heater going full blast, we adjourned to the shooting range.

I loaded my trusty S&W .357 with the brand-spanking new ammo I'd purchased and faced the bad guy snarling at me from the fluttering paper clipped to a wooden frame. The range was about five yards.

"Isn't this a little close?" I asked the instructor.

"We ain't teachin' you to be a sniper. Most gunfights are up close and personal."

Chastened, I fired off my six rounds with the rest of my shivering companions. We advanced to the targets. Not bad. All were grouped fairly tightly in the center mass. Of course the S&W sported a 6" barrel, allowing me to practically touch the target with the muzzle. Still, I felt the spirit of Wyatt Earp stir within me. Just a little.

We increased the distance and practiced shooting while moving from side to side. I'm proud to say I didn't shoot any of my fellow students even once. Daylight was fading early in the gray sky when our instructor called a halt and led us back to the shack. We all got certificates and broke for the warmth of our cars.

I don't know about Denise, but I got to thinking about when and where I'd carry a concealed weapon. I couldn't take it into work, and I wasn't crazy about wearing a gun around the house, concealed or not. In the end the .357 went back in its file drawer with the ammunition stored at the other end of the house. If someone's coming to get me, I'll need at least fifteen minutes notice.

Sixteen

Family Ties

It's a cliché that when a person goes to jail, his whole family goes with him. It's certainly a traumatic time for everyone, but it's often easier for the jail staff to deal with the prisoner than the family on the outside. Sometimes it feels like the whole family's been arrested, or should be.

Arthur Garmin was arrested due to his wife, Beatrice's, complaint of domestic violence. Arthur beat Beatrice on a regular basis, and the neighbors could count on a visit from the police sometime every weekend. The arrest reports were monotonous in quoting Beatrice's shouted grievances against her worthless husband.

Arthur had high blood pressure, which he took great pride in ignoring. On his admission to CJC, the intake nurse noted a pressure of 180/110—stroke territory. He was taken to medical for evaluation. His pressure came down a little after passing through the booking procedure, but it still ranged around 160/100. I asked Arthur if he'd like to change his mind and take some medication to bring it down.

Arthur was still angry with the police interference in his private matters and told me curtly to fuck off. That's his privilege. I warned him about his persistent hypertension, but he just snorted and demanded to be taken to his housing pod. That night Arthur had a stroke, which left him paralyzed on the left side.

This much was predictable. It was only a matter of when it was going to happen. Still, you never want it to happen on your watch when there was such a good chance to correct it fairly simply.

Beatrice went ballistic. Arthur was her knight in shining armor, her pole star, her hero. And now he lay in a hospital bed drooling out the corner of his mouth, unable to even walk to the bathroom. Beatrice did the only thing she could. She sued the sheriff for negligence and deliberate indifference to her sainted husband's obvious needs.

Long story short, Arthur and Beatrice collected eighty-five grand and lived comparatively happily ever after, since Arthur couldn't effectively beat her up anymore. It's good to have a compassionate family looking out for your best interests.

Often it's Mom that gets involved. I thought this was something exclusive to prison inmates, but it turns out to be pretty universal.

I was sitting in Denise's office going over Director of Nursing stuff when Wendy, our HSA, poked her head in. She pointed to Denise's phone. "Take this," she snarled through clenched teeth. "I can't take it anymore."

Wendy stomped back to her office and a moment later Denise's phone lit up. "This likely isn't someone notifying you that you've won the lottery," I said, starting to get up.

Denise waved me back to my chair. "We'll share," she said and punched the speaker button. "This is Denise."

"Denise who?" the speaker demanded.

"I'm the Director of Nursing. Who am I speaking with?"

"This is Rodney's mother. Where's that other woman?"

"Our administrator had to leave for a moment and thought I might be able to help you."

"Bullshit. She hung up on me. I know what you're doing to Rodney."

"Lower your voice, Mrs.—may I have your last name?"

"I already been through all that with that other woman."

"I understand, but I need to know your son's name so I can look up his file."

"Rodney. His name is Rodney. R-O-D-N-E-Y. Rodney. Are you people all stupid?"

"A last name, please."

"Phillips, as you already well know."

"Thank you, Mrs. Phillips, now what—"

"Phillips is not my name. My name is Archer. Phillips is Rodney's name."

"Okay, Mrs. Archer. Now what seems to be the problem?"

"Rodney needs his pain medicine. Why aren't you giving him his pain medicine?"

"Let me see what—"

"You been keeping his medicine. He needs that medicine. Rodney got pain."

"I see on his intake sheet that he was taking Percocet for ankle pain."

"That's right. He be taking that for a couple of years. He need that medicine."

"Percocet is a narcotic, Mrs. Archer. We don't allow narcotics here at CJC."

"Rodney in terrific pain. He told me so. You need to give him that medicine."

"Just a second, Mrs. Archer." Denise put her on hold and called the housing pod. She spoke briefly and got back to Rodney's mother.

"I just checked with the deputy on his housing unit, Mrs. Archer. She told me Rodney is playing basketball."

"Well, he got to exercise."

"If Rodney has a problem with his ankle, he can send a kite to medical, and one of our providers would be glad to look at him. Sorry, we can't allow Percocet in here."

"You all the same. You be hearing from Rodney's lawyer."

"I'll look forward to it, Mrs. Archer. Have a nice day."

It seemed universal. Whenever a prisoner wanted something, he didn't put in a kite for the doctor, he didn't contact his lawyer, he called Mom. We got a lot of calls from moms about how their sons were being mistreated, and they always were very sincere. Mom believed her son unquestioningly despite his past performances and was hell-bent to take up his cause.

I can appreciate a mother's love for her offspring, but nearly always she's been taken in by his one-sided spin. She's so used to his lies that a few more don't make much difference.

Fortunately for me, I didn't have to talk to Mom very often. Usually the administration fielded these calls unless there was a real medical issue at stake. Like my ulcerative colitis patient, Scott. Scott's mom wanted to know why her son wasn't on his UC medication.

"Scott didn't mention taking any medication for his UC. He said it hasn't flared up in over a year."

"That's not true. I give him money for his medication every month. He's regular with it."

"You get the medicine for him?"

"No, I can't get out. I give him money for it, and he gets it. Pretty expensive too. Is that why you aren't giving it to him?"

"No, ma'am. I'm not giving it to him because he doesn't need it. Do you think Scott might have taken the money and not bought medicine with it?"

"I knew you'd say something like that. My Scotty's a good boy."

"Is that why he's in jail for the third time?"

"Quack!"

"Is that a request or an opinion?" I have some clever stock answers ready for such occasions.

<click>

SEVENTEEN

ADVENTURES IN MEDICAL

Seeing patients in my medical clinic was pretty much like seeing them in private practice except for the patients. Stacy, my medical assistant, triaged the kites in order of perceived urgency and piled them on my schedule along with patients scheduled because of diseases that needed chronic attention, like diabetes or high blood pressure.

This mélange of illnesses was picked up by deputies one housing pod at a time. They trooped down in a line to the medical waiting room, a cell the size of a smallish office just off the main corridor. There was a matching cell across from the waiting area cell for people who had finished their appointments and were gathering for the return trip.

It wasn't always set up like this. We used to have males on one side of the corridor and females on the other. We have an inmate bathroom just down the hall.

One of the women needed to use the facilities and asked a staff member to let her go. No problem. A few minutes later one of the men asked a different staff member for the same privilege.

Imagine the shock when an aide opened the bathroom door five minutes later to see what was taking the man so long. The two lovers were caught in flagrante delicto and promptly pried apart.

Being locked up in jail is an impediment to communication between the sexes, but to the determined that hardly matters. Napoleon, who spent some time behind bars himself, said, "Circumstances—what are circumstances? I make circumstances."

A peculiarity in the CJC plumbing makes it possible for females in Alpha to talk to males in Charlie via the toilets. Talk about romance. Just don't flush at the wrong moment.

A Muslim inmate working in the kitchen sent messages to his love via a sandwich on a special Muslim diet tray. He'd get her reply by looking in a potato chip bag on her returning tray. Worked like a charm for months until he got transferred.

In prisons and jails there is no such thing as consensual sex. Every instance is treated as a rape, even a situation like the two lovers in medical's bathroom. Maybe the man had threatened the woman to set this encounter up. Maybe it was the woman's idea. There are lots of ways that an inmate of either sex could be intimidated. Since there's really no way to know for sure, there's a zero tolerance policy.

Currently there's a big push for the precepts of the Prison Rape Elimination Act (PREA). These are procedures designed to analyze the incidence of rape in prisons and jails and to come up with ways to eliminate it.

The problem isn't trivial. Because of methodological problems, studies of the prevalence of rape in institutions give widely disparate values. We don't really know how commonly rape and sexual harassment occur.

It's safe to say that many people, including inmates, view incarceration as a recipe for rape, but it's not at all clear that it's true. Any rape is abhorrent, but to think of prisons and jails as hotbeds of fornication is overstating what really happens. Yes, people have sex in prisons, but it seems that most is consensual and therefore non-violent.

It's especially a problem for the gay and trans-gender inmates who are more often targets for exploitation. Sex offenders are also low men on the totem pole of jail status. Colorado prisons deal with this partially by concentrating like with like, but the jails have less flexibility because of housing constraints. There are only so many places to put people.

It doesn't matter. The zero-tolerance policy mandates that prison and jail staff do all they can to shut down incidents of rape or sexual harassment. The motivation of the participants, while important to them, is beside the point for security staff. I'm good with that.

I became intimately acquainted with the zero tolerance policy via Gary Hanson, a middle-aged pedophile. I knew something was up when Sergeant Gomez, a member of the internal investigative team at CJC, casually stopped by my office.

"Got a minute, Doc?"

"Sure. What's up?"

"Mind if I shut the door?"

"Sure." I was getting a bad feeling about this.

"How do you usually examine patients?"

"For what?"

"Well, for anything. Like you're doing a physical or something."

I described what a physical exam consisted of and pantomimed the actions. "That cover it?" I asked.

"You get close to the patients?"

"Sure, right next to them. Listening to the heart and lungs, feeling the abdomen. What's all this about?"

Gomez didn't answer, but asked, "How close?"

"Next to them. Then exam table's narrow and I'm right up against it sometimes."

"So you touch them?"

"Of course. Hands on the shoulder. Hands on the back. Leaning over. How else am I supposed to do a physical exam? It's not something you do across the room. That's why they call it physical."

He pointed to the entry. "You keep the door open all the time?"

"Door's open unless I'm having a private phone conversation. There's a drape I can pull so folks in the hall don't have to watch something gross."

"Somebody in here with you?"

"Stacy's usually here, but unless the patient's a female, she's in and out. She also works with Gloria next door. Ready to tell me what this is all about?"

Gomez looked slightly embarrassed. "You remember Gary Hanson?"

"Can't say that I do. Hold on a second and I'll look him up." I turned to the computer and brought up his record. The head and shoulders picture of a heavy-set, partly balding man popped onto the screen. "Hmm. I don't remember him particularly. Why? What's the problem?"

"He says you raped him," Gomez deadpanned.

"You're kidding."

"Nope. Says you touched him inappropriately while you were alone here in the room with him."

I looked through the electronic record of what was a routine physical exam. "Bullshit."

"Hey, Doc, I have to ask. I've got to take every complaint seriously."

"I'm on Medicare," I said. "I'm a little past raping age."

"Whatever," Gomez said, spreading his hands in a helpless gesture.

I pointed to the picture. "He's not that good-looking. Do you think this is the best candidate I could come up with?"

"Just my job, Doc. Can you come with me?"

"You're kidding."

He wasn't. We trooped down to his office and into a soundproof room with a table and two straight chairs. Something that looked like a laptop computer sat on the table.

"What's that?" I asked.

"Stress analysis," Gomez replied, setting some switches. "Routine."

"A lie detector."

"Sorry, Doc, I got to ask you some questions."

For those of you unfamiliar with voice stress analysis (VSA), it works by analyzing "microtremors" in speech, which are supposedly produced by the subject attempting to deceive the questioner. There aren't any wires or pen recorder prints like a traditional polygraph lie detector. The entire setup is a laptop computer running the VSA program, and a microphone.

There's lots of controversy about VSA, with several studies showing that it's no more accurate than flipping a coin. The polygraph community hates it, but lots of law enforcement agencies use it because it's simple and cheap. Then again, so is flipping a nickel.

Gomez started out with some baseline questions.

"Just answer yes or no, Doc," he said. "Is your name William Wright?"

"Yes."

"Is today Tuesday?"

"No."

"Is today Wednesday?"

"Yes."

"Are we in Colorado Springs?"

"Yes."

"Did you do a physical examination on Gary Hanson?"

"Yes."

"Are you sitting in a chair?"

"Yes."

"Did you touch Mr. Hanson inappropriately during the exam?"

"No."

"Is there a table in this room?"

"Yes."

"Did you touch Mr. Hanson's genitals during the exam?"

"No."

"Did you make sexual comments to Mr. Hanson during the exam?"

"No."

"Is there a microphone on the table?"

"Yes."

"Did you have an erection during your examination of Mr. Hanson?"

"No."

Permutations of this went on for a while, going from baseline questions to pointed references to fondling Hanson's nether regions. Suffice to say, the interview was thorough. It was surreal to think that Gomez or anyone else could take these charges seriously, but on reflection I could see that they had to. More than once I thought I should be calling a lawyer. At length we finished.

I looked at Gomez. "So?"

"We'll be in touch," he said noncommittally.

"Did I pass?" I persisted.

"We'll be in touch."

Two weeks later Gomez sidled into my office again. "It's all good, Doc," he said and left.

I never found out what Hanson had in mind with his accusation. It was the only time I'd seen him, so I hadn't had time to piss him off. He hadn't asked for anything out of the ordinary at his exam, so that didn't seem to be the motivation. Maybe he was a friend of somebody who held a grudge. Since I'm strikingly handsome and personable, maybe I was his fantasy lover. I'll never know. All I know is that Hanson is off my clinic list forever.

Doctors are taught from early medical school days about respecting the bodies of our patients. It's even in the Hippocratic Oath we take. I've always been conscious about having a chaperone while examining a female patient, but I'll admit I let my guard down with the less-than-hygienic males I see. I'd be more likely to attack them with a can of Lysol than try to rape one of them.

The jail is a tough venue for modesty. I can't have a medical assistant or other warm body in the room with me all the time. There's not enough staff as it is to do the work, let alone assigning someone to be an official chaperone. Ah well, at my age I guess I should be flattered.

Where there's testosterone, there's sex, and we've got plenty of the former. Sadly, the inmates aren't the only ones who participate. Sometimes it's the fox guarding the henhouse.

One scandal involved two deputies who worked a tag team with some of the female inmates. After things had settled down for the night, the pair would select their companion for the evening and escort her down to the laundry facility. One would function as lookout while the other entertained the lady.

It worked for a while until someone got suspicious about these late night transports and started reviewing the camera tapes. Oops.

Men aren't always the instigators. A female deputy was walked out of the facility after security discovered she was servicing a number of the male inmates. Apparently she was picky about who she chose, and she was turned in by the males she rejected. Who can you trust anymore?

The path of true love is never smooth. A CJC nurse took a shine to an inmate on the third tier. Since she had keys to the housing pod doors, she started meeting him in the recreation area for extracurricular activities.

Even though she had the keys, she forgot about the cameras. She was busted and walked out of the facility. She didn't give up though. She divorced her husband, a deputy at CJC, and waited for her true love to get out of the clink. They married and had a child. We'll wait to see how this turns out. He was in for domestic violence.

Not to leave those of alternate persuasion out of the litany, a gay food service supervisor was busted for giving and receiving oral sex in the kitchen cooler. Disgruntled snitches put a stop to that. It's yet another reason I brown bag it a lot.

I see instances of rape infrequently, certainly less than I see in the community at large. We try to minimize the opportunities by the choice of housing pod and whether known sexual predators are allowed near other prisoners. We can also house particularly vulnerable inmates in medical if needed.

Those people that we do house in medical are a diverse lot. These are folks who aren't sick enough to go to the hospital, but are too sick to go back into general population. You'll find inmates who are coming back from surgery or from a stay in the hospital for pneumonia or kidney failure. Out-of-control diabetics or people with casts are frequent visitors. We don't allow most casts or braces on the housing pods, especially if they contain any metal. Taking a cast or brace apart to make a shiv out of the metal reinforcing strip is too easy.

One patient, who wanted to get out of the isolation of a medical cell, beat his arm cast against the cell wall until it literally disintegrated. I examined him, judged that if the arm could stand up to that beating it was probably healed enough, and sent him back to the housing pod.

We kept people in medical who required ongoing specialized nursing care. One patient had hidden from the cops high in the Colorado mountains. By the time he was caught, he'd gotten a good case of frostbite on his feet. His wound care featured auto-amputation of his toes, which fell off like raisins with dressing changes. Sorry, it's gross I know, but if you're a medical type it's something you don't see every day.

Hepatitis C is a blood-borne disease popular with inmates who get tattoos or use IV drugs. Hep C leads to liver cirrhosis, which leads to bleeding from veins in the esophagus. Vomiting up a bellyful of blood is not the best way to start your day. I saw a lot of folks coming back from having these veins banded to shut off the bleeding.

These residents of our clinic often played cute tricks on the nursing staff. A favorite was to pile poop by the cell door. When the nurse came in to take vital signs in the morning… Hilarity of the first order.

We had one patient who loved to dance. Every time anyone came near his cell he'd jump up and start doing a hula complete with arm waving and bump-and-grind. Fascinating.

Usually, inmates occupied individual cells in medical as opposed to sharing a room in general population. One inmate with a persistent oral infection kept the ball rolling by packing a tooth with feces to keep it infected so he could stay in his own private room.

We had to monitor inmates on hunger strikes. We could watch and monitor them until they got loopy, then we could legally intervene with IVs and forced feedings via a tube inserted through the nose into the stomach. Also gross, but usually one trip through this procedure was enough to convince the striker to give it up.

One hunger-striker was perplexing. Instead of losing weight, he was actually gaining. Long story short, his attorney was bringing him McDonalds during meetings at the courthouse. Now that's the way to do a hunger strike.

EIGHTEEN

CHECKING OUT

Most of the inmates at CJC would rather be somewhere else. Fortunately, most prisoners only stayed at the jail a short time, but many were on their way to extended incarceration in Colorado's prison system. For repeat offenders—the norm, it seemed—heading down that road again is too much to take, and the only way they saw out was suicide.

Fear, shame, and anger are normal emotions in jail, but loneliness is probably the most powerful. The new inmate has to learn how to survive in this foreign milieu of disparate groups, who to trust, who to avoid, and how to interact with all of them. A major issue is just having a sense of purpose, the ability to look beyond the present situation. Some fail at this.

Hanging is the most prevalent avenue, and security is tasked with preventing this by observing inmates and making frequent rounds to check that everyone's still alive. Even this isn't enough if someone is determined enough.

I've mentioned Terrance, a guy who swan-dived to the concrete from the second tier and Angela, a woman who got a free trip to the hospital with a faked suicide attempt. There's more.

A young lady was found on morning rounds hanging from an upper bunk, sitting Indian-style on the lower bunk with a book open in her lap. She'd been dead for about eight hours without the deputy noticing, despite rounding every fifteen minutes. You'd think that reading a book in a cell with no lights would have raised some suspicions. Mental health had cleared the inmate as having no issues. Oops. The deputy was fired and mental health got a rap on the knuckles. They finally decided she was suffering from post-partum depression. No kidding.

Another woman jumped from the second tier, a popular launching place, and fell on a six-months-pregnant woman below. Both survived, and the pregnant woman didn't abort. In a twist, the jumper was in for killing her newborn child.

Not trusting the fall to kill him, a man jumped from the second tier with a sheet wrapped around his neck and tied to the top rail. He was caught by inmates below and held aloft until the sheet could be untied. No plan is perfect.

Another man waited until the deputy on the pod looked up before he acted. He had a sheet around his neck like the other jumper. He waved a cheery good-bye to the deputy and then jumped from the second tier. The deputy miraculously got under him and caught him, holding him up until the sheet could be cut loose.

In another episode, a nurse discovered an inmate hanging in his cell. The deputies, following protocol, began to leave to put together a team. The nurse, seeing the man was still alive, rushed in and held him up, relieving the pressure on the noose.

There's a good reason for putting the entry team together. More than one prisoner has faked an injury to lure staff into his cell so he could attack them. Still, standing there and watching a man strangle to death goes against the grain, especially for us medical types.

However, no good deed goes unpunished. The nurse was brought up on charges for violating the jail protocol by entering the cell alone. The prisoner sued her for aborting his suicide attempt. Only in America.

While not really a suicide attempt, the production of alcoholic beverages in jails has some decidedly lethal propensities. The traditional concoction, Pruno, comes from combining any manner of sugar-containing substrate like fruit with yeast and letting the mixture sit in a warm place for as long as you can stand the smell.

The mixture, contained in a plastic soft-drink bottle, has a gelatinous top layer of bread, the source of the yeast, and a swampy bottom layer of fruit rinds with a hazy liquid in between. Taking the top from a bottle releases a smell powerful enough to knock over a rhino.

To avoid all the smell, mess, and horrible taste of Pruno, inmates sometimes can score a bottle of hand sanitizer from the offices they visit. Hand sanitizer is mostly ethyl alcohol. The one sitting on my desk is 70 percent ethanol, 140 proof. It's the other 30 percent that'll get you.

Putting salt in the sanitizer will separate the alcohol from the gel. The problem is, the ethanol is denatured. What this means is that other stuff is put in to make the alcohol undrinkable.

Methanol or methyl alcohol isn't used in hand sanitizers because not only is it toxic, but it can be absorbed through the skin. Isopropyl alcohol, rubbing alcohol, isn't absorbed as much and is indeed used in hand sanitizers. I see it on the label of mine.

Isopropyl alcohol is toxic if you drink it, but it's likely that the imbiber wouldn't be able to tell the toxicity from the effects of getting drunk until he goes blind or gets brain, liver or kidney failure. Some that drink this mixture don't have to wait for organ failure. They die from acute alcohol poisoning from drinking too much of the high proof ethanol.

Not all the danger is to the consumer. Victor Reales was brought in recently on a homicide charge with a medical twist. It seems he was drinking vodka, mouthwash, and hand sanitizer early one morning with one of his buddies and suddenly decided to bludgeon him to death with a rock. There's a lesson in here somewhere.

Not all jail inmates get out via suicide. Most are released on bond, acquitted of charges, or simply serve their time and leave. What happens when I run into my former patients at Wal-Mart?

Not much. For one thing, I don't necessarily travel in the same circles as my patients, but if I do run into one on the outside, things are pretty cordial. Some are kind of embarrassed and shy, but manage to say hello. Some are more enthusiastic and greet me like an old buddy. *Hey, Doc, remember when you treated that rash I had at CJC?*

Well, I usually don't remember, but I'm always glad to see them in better circumstances. Sometimes they're with their families, and I get introduced around. Probably the ones who hate my guts are waiting in the parking lot.

NINETEEN

INFAMOUS INMATES

Maria Dixon was twenty-five years old when she doused her five children with gasoline and set them on fire. She later said she was depressed after her husband committed suicide three months earlier. Someone should have noticed a few screws loose when she asked the funeral home to have her husband stuffed. She wanted to prop him up on the couch so they could watch TV together forever. The undertaker declined.

As her apartment burned with her five children, Dixon inflicted a few superficial cuts on her arms and ran for it. When apprehended, she blamed lack of attention from a social worker for making her incinerate her kids.

When she was incarcerated at CJC awaiting trial, Dixon turned into a drama queen every time the dressings were changed on her arm cuts, wailing and complaining about her severe pain. The professionalism of the nurses was severely tested and I'm afraid my disgust showed.

Ultimately Dixon was sentenced to eighty-five years in the Colorado Women's Prison, where she gave TV interviews about how distraught she was over the loss of her children. She managed to be tearful when claiming it never would have happened if only the social worker had taken her children away before she could hurt them.

Teenage angst came to the fore with Daniel Forrester. Daniel, aged fifteen, was living with his grandmother. Like many teenagers, he chafed at the terminal embarrassment of having his grandmother drive him to school.

One morning he took the only option he could think of by tiptoeing into her room, placing a shotgun on her sleeping face and pulling the trigger. A withdrawn teen, he had no medical problems for me to address, but he was treated by the mental health staff at CJC before continuing into the prison population. The last I heard of him was the argument over whether he should be tried as an adult, but by that time he'd passed out of my orbit.

Tim and Deb Porter were living the high life selling methamphetamine to the Colorado Springs trade. Their mistake was to begin using their own product. Bills mounted and the couple found themselves in deep with their suppliers.

What better way to raise some cash than to heavily insure their three children and hope for an accident? Tim and Deb weren't disposed to wait for natural occurrences, so they poured gasoline on the kids and torched their apartment for the combined insurance payoff.

Things didn't work out well for the couple. They left tons of evidence for the arson investigators and instead of a suite in the Bahamas, they got a couple of cells at CJC. They were pissed at being caught, but unrepentant otherwise. Despite public anguish over the deaths of their children, in the confines of the jail they remained arrogant, indifferent, and nasty. After a stint at CJC, they graduated to life without parole in Colorado prisons.

It's proven hard for me to treat monsters like these. It's one of the big reasons I preferred not to know the offenses of my patients. In general these people were quite similar to the ones I treated in Colorado State Penitentiary, the state's maximum-security prison.

They usually had no empathy for their victims and no real appreciation that they'd done something wrong. They tended to be very narcissistic with a constant aura of entitlement. I had a hard time maintaining professional objectivity and found myself avoiding any contact that wasn't absolutely mandatory. That's not good when you're the only doctor available, but I have to give myself the pass of being human too.

One of the most horrendous cases came through the jail before I got there. George Woldt and Lucas Salmon, both 23 years old, snatched Jacine Gielinski, a 22-year-old University of Colorado at Colorado Springs coed, off the street. They drove to an elementary school parking lot where they took turns raping her. They then slit her throat, stabbed her in the chest and smothered her. Finally they shoved mud into her vagina to cover up

DNA evidence, tossed her nude body under a van, and exchanged "high fives"

Salmon got life without parole. Woldt, the instigator of the whole business, was sentenced by a panel of three judges to the death penalty. His defense attorneys argued that he should be spared because he had a brain lesion that impaired his judgment, he has obsessive-compulsive disorder, he was abused as a child, and he had become a Christian since he was incarcerated. Oh, please.

Woldt was likely one of my patients when I was the physician at Colorado State Penitentiary. That's where all the death row inmates reside, but I don't remember seeing him. Just as well.

Woldt lucked out, sort of, with a commuted sentence to life without parole after the U.S. Supreme Court ruled that the judges couldn't give him the death penalty. That had to be done by a jury. Now he's out on the eastern plains of Colorado at Limon Correctional Facility.

Nolan Samuels, a 34-year-old redneck, stepped in front of an 18-wheeler and got squashed like a bug on the windshield. A sheriff's deputy got to him and kept the pieces together until they got him to the hospital. He survived, but, as they say, "was never quite the same again."

He began a life of crime and, as amateurs will, he made mistakes. He was arrested on burglary charges and met up with the deputy who saved his life at CJC. Nolan wasn't all that grateful, and became a behavior problem.

It seems after the accident he was pretty much impervious to pain of any sort. Probably used it all up. Also, he couldn't stand to be in a cell next to anyone else.

The El Paso County Courthouse has holding cells in the basement for prisoners awaiting their turn before the judge. As you might imagine, it's a depressing place with cinderblock walls and barred doors.

When it was Nolan's turn to go to the courthouse for his hearing, there was another prisoner in the cell next to him. Nolan started punching the common wall of the two cells, actually taking chunks out of the concrete with his fists trying to get to the guy next to him. The only thing that saved the day was a good dose of pepper spray.

We had an inmate, Georgio Pappandreas, who was a former member of the Greek Olympic wrestling team. No kidding. He was a little past his prime, but still imposing. When it was time for him to go downtown to court, he decided he didn't want to go.

In a quick series of moves that would bring tears to the eyes of any civil rights activist, the SWAT team suited up and confronted the poised Geogio. No contest. He was doused with pepper spray, subdued by six heavily-padded attackers, had his clothes cut off, carried upside-down to the showers, re-clothed, and off to court in four-point restraints before you can say, "Opa!"

One of my colleagues in another jail told me about how he dealt with an inmate who constantly came to his clinic demanding narcotics for neck pain. The man was arrested for a particularly brutal double murder of his wife and her paramour.

It seems he had discovered the couple, gone to his workshop and retrieved a crowbar, which he then used to almost decapitate both of the lovers. My friend related part of his clinic visit.

"You got to give me something stronger for this, Doc. My neck. I can't hardly stand it."

"The neck pain's really bad, is it?"

"Horrible."

"Is this like sort of a crampy kind of neck pain or more like a crowbar in the neck kind?"

The inmate cussed him out and stomped out of the clinic.

One of the most horrific rape and assault cases occurred here in August of 2012. A 53-year-old woman who worked nights was checking her mail at 1:30 in the morning. She heard two groups of men arguing in the parking lot of her apartment and intervened, convincing the belligerents to cool off rather than fight.

Afterwards, one of the men invited her back to his apartment as thanks. She drank what she believed to be lemonade in a room with five Iraqi men in their twenties and doesn't remember anything after that.

What happened was a rectal and oral rape that nearly killed her from internal bleeding. One of the primary aggressors was a man named Ramadon. He was notable for being featured in a combat memoir, *A Soldier's Promise,* by Army First Sergeant Daniel Hendrex. In the book Hendrex describes how Ramadon, then fourteen, helped American troops fighting in Iraq by passing along information about forty insurgents, including his own terrorist father. In exchange, Hendrex helped Ramadon immigrate to the United States. They were even on Oprah.

The Iraqis were held in medical at CJC because of the danger that they would be killed in the housing pods. Ramadon, a muscular 21-year-old with close-cropped hair and dark, hooded eyes gazing impassively from a blocky head, complained that he wanted a special diet. He wanted pain medicine for muscle aches. He wanted a special exercise period. He had a bruise that required immediate attention. His hand hurt and he wanted an x-ray. It was probably the one he used in the rectal rape.

Like the other monsters I'd treated, it was all about him. He never expressed anything but contempt for the nurses, the women who should be serving him and catering to his desires. I never heard a word of remorse for the good Samaritan whom he'd ravaged and almost killed.

He didn't get any extra falafel from me.

TWENTY

DANGER IS MY BUSINESS

People ask me if working in a prison or jail is dangerous. Well, yeah, but it's probably safer than something like hard rock mining or servicing high voltage power lines. It's really safe enough if you pay attention to where you are and what you're doing.

For the most part, the patients I saw were already in enough trouble and didn't want to add to it. That doesn't mean you let your guard down and get sloppy. Some were looking at so much jail and prison time that they didn't care. They felt they had nothing to lose. You can't fall out of the basement.

The tactic that's always worked for me is first to be aware of the situation I'm in. If I'm isolated in a room with an inmate between me and the only exit, that's not good. If I'm walking ahead of an inmate to the exam room, that's not good either. It's a no-no to leave a blunt instrument like an otoscope within easy reach of the inmate. If I feel anger or even irritation with an inmate, it's time to wrap up the visit.

One of my predecessor medical directors apparently forgot this precept. Although she was a tiny woman, she was famous for getting in the inmates' faces with her irritation. One time she picked the wrong guy to disrespect. He launched across the exam room and cleaned her clock before the deputies could intervene. I heard she was a little more restrained after that.

So was I afraid of my patients? No. There were enough safeguards on my side that I didn't worry much about that. Did I trust them? Not in a million years. While some might have come to Jesus and transformed into a model citizens, I wouldn't leave my wallet or an extra syringe on the desk.

As much as I'd like to deny it, jails and prisons are dangerous places. It's more dangerous for the inmates than for me, but there are enough instances of inmates assaulting or killing staff members for me to keep my guard up.

Although I haven't been physically assaulted in the jail, I get threatened on a regular basis. Elton Delgado showed up in my clinic wanting a lower bunk restriction.

"I can't get up on the top bunk, Doc." He held out a limp wrist for inspection. "It hurts too much when I have to hold the ladder. I really need a lower bunk."

"What's the trouble with your wrist?" I asked, bringing up his medical record on the computer.

"I was in this motorcycle accident. Screwed it up." He winced with the recollection, cradling his right wrist in his left palm for support.

"I don't see anything about an injury here in the record. When did this happen?"

"Couple of years ago. It was in California." Funny how when I need information, it's always in another state.

"What doctor did you see?"

"Some guy in the emergency room. I don't remember his name."

"This emergency room, where was it?"

"Some little town east of Sacramento I think. San something-or-other."

"Ah, San something-or-other. A great place."

"Yeah. Can I get this lower bunk?"

I examined the hand, finding nothing wrong other than Elton's protestations of pain. I could see the calluses on his palms and fingers. A basketball player.

"I think you're good, Mr. Delgado. No need to restrict you to a lower bunk."

He looked at me open-mouthed, uncomprehending. "You're kidding."

"Nope. Wrist is okay. You're good to go."

"Motherfucker," he muttered.

Most of the time I ignore these *sotto voce* insults unless the inmate is looking at me when he says it. In that case it's personal and I can't let it pass. If I did, there would be more and more in-your-face exchanges coming up with inmates thinking they could browbeat and insult the medical providers whenever they felt like it.

I paused from my typing and looked Elton in the face, holding his gaze. "What was that?" I asked.

Most of the time this elicits a scowl, averted eyes and a sullen, mumbled, "Nuthin'." Fine. We can all go about our business. Elton didn't take this option.

His mouth hardened into a line. "You heard me," he said.

I nodded. "I did." I called to the deputy outside the door. "Sergeant, could you escort Mr. Delgado to the SHU?"

"Motherfucker!" Delgado shouted. "You can't stick me in the fucking SHU!"

The deputy grabbed Delgado's shoulder. "I can, and I just did. Come back when you can control your mouth."

I've found that if I take care of negative situations quickly and consistently, pretty soon the inmates know what they can and can't do in medical in general, and with me in particular. I'm not sure how I'd handle it if I didn't have a cadre of burly deputies handy, but that's one of the perks of the job.

What about when an inmate gets out of jail? Am I worried that he's going to come after me or my family? I haven't experienced anything like this, likely because the freed prisoners have other things to worry about like eating and finding shelter. Still, I keep in mind people like my old patient at Colorado State Penitentiary, Evan Ebel, who got out and murdered Colorado prisons director Tom Clements at his home.

When Ebel was gunned down by Texas lawmen, a hit list with twenty more names was found in his car. Investigations indicate that the assassination list originated with the 211 Crew command structure rather than Ebel acting alone. It happens, but I can't let the possibility make me hide under the bed when I go home.

The subject came up fairly frequently at home when I first started to work in corrections. My wife, Mollie, an inveterate watcher of true crime shows, kept expecting a low rider packed with gun-toting vigilantes to come cruising up our street looking for revenge. Not yet.

How I feel personally about an inmate shouldn't enter into the conversation about his medical problems. He's not in jail so I can give him more grief. It's well to keep in mind that although these people may have made bad choices to get here, it doesn't mean they should be treated with less respect than any other patient.

This is not just altruism. If I treat a person with respect, it's more likely that he'll reciprocate. Respect is the oil that makes the whole machine run better. If I don't show that respect, I can look forward to more conflict and poor medical outcomes. If someone thinks I'm a jerk, they aren't very likely to follow my medical program. If I think he's a jerk, well, that's my problem.

It's my job to be the best doctor I can be for them, not to be an instrument of their punishment. I'll admit that it's a hard thing to accomplish for some of the arrogant gangbangers, child molesters, or the perpetrators of the more egregious crimes. Still, it's the job I signed up for back when I took the Hippocratic Oath. I'm supposed to be a healer, not a judge.

TWENTY-ONE

LOST AND FOUND

The thing about contraband is that inmates aren't supposed to have it. Does that stop them? It does not. Inmates are endlessly inventive when it comes to acquisition of illegal substances.

First in line are drugs. We'd like to think that jails would be places where drugs are rare. Not so. There are barriers to drug trafficking, but the barriers are more like sieves than solid walls. So how do the drugs get in?

The most common avenue is through visitors. The more liberal the visitation rules of a facility, the more easily drugs are introduced into the system.

A kiss is an opportunity to pass a heroin balloon mouth-to-mouth. A handshake conceals the transfer of a packet of cocaine. A chocolate bar or cup of coffee hides the narcotic package underneath.

How do the visitors carry the drugs in? After all, everyone is subject to searches. Concealment in body cavities is common. A quick trip to the restroom allows extraction of a package from the vagina or rectum. This includes larger items like cell phones and chargers, even knives (carefully wrapped). One lady visitor with a more-than-ample derriere had a stash of drugs taped to her behind. Well-endowed visitors can secrete all manner of items in their bras.

Some corpulent visitors hide drugs in their bellybuttons. Underwear is popular as a location where searches tend to be cursory at best. Even Little Goo is suspect. Many jails require infants to have diapers opened before admission. Lawyers, bless their hearts, have been known to smuggle drugs in legal papers, supposedly immune from search.

Sad to say, another major source of contraband is the prison staff. Motivated by sex, money or intimidation, it's relatively easy for a deputy or jail worker to smuggle items in. It's simple to put a cell phone between two pieces of bread or pills inside a soda can. Even more easily than visitors, jail staff can smuggle items in body cavities.

I'm a pack rat. At CJC I didn't once get searched while carrying in a black gym bag stuffed with books, rubber exercise bands, reading glasses, folders of articles, a flurry of loose papers, my frozen lunch du jour, a stethoscope case, and a partridge. Smuggling would have been a cinch.

The mail is a great avenue as well. Dots of black tar heroin under a stamp, a greeting card saturated with methamphetamine, or a cute drawing from a daughter with "To Daddy" scrawled across the paper smeared with a nearly invisible layer of narcotic or LSD all arrive in the mail to brighten the day of the poor prisoner.

Although not such a problem at CJC because of the enclosed structure, a tried-and-true method of introducing contraband into a jail is simply to throw it over the wall into a common area. Contraband cell phones are used to set up an appointment for delivery with a precisely timed pseudo-fight as a diversion. Tennis balls slit open and stuffed with pills are easy when public roads or houses are close to prison walls. One enterprising jail employee brought in two footballs filled with cigarettes, marijuana, pills, cell phones and chargers, which she planned on leaving in the recreation area.

For more distance, bows and arrows can fill the bill with the bonus of introducing a weapon along with the drug cargo. Paintball guns or homemade "spud guns" serve as launching platforms as well. More recently technology enables delivery of contraband by mini-helicopter drones controlled anonymously at long distance. This is an improvement on the previous carrier pigeon delivery method, as the birds frequently flew off course.

Pigeons still have their uses. A variation on the tennis ball ploy is to put the contraband inside a dead pigeon and heave it over the wall. Supposedly this is not as suspicious to find in the common area.

Other prisoners are part of the contraband chain. A trusted prisoner working at an off-prison site can acquire the contraband and carry it back to the dealer. A trusted prisoner might have his wife or girlfriend bring in contraband to a visit. She transfers it to the trusted prisoner, who later passes it to the final recipient. This way the prisoner under suspicion can have a clean visitor and be clean himself before and after the visit.

Some jails have policies that allow inmates to receive food items from outside. You can see this one coming. A jar of olives with the pimentos replaced by little red heroin balloons. A jar of peanut butter, microwaved to make it smooth, concealing a cargo of cocaine. Even a pizza whose layer of cheese concealed a layer of heroin.

Heroin remains the drug of choice. Cocaine is relatively expensive, and the high is short-lived—perhaps forty-five minutes on average. Heroin, on the other hand, will last much longer—up to nine or ten hours at a time. It's also easily hidden. A dose of black tar heroin is about the size of the period at the end of this sentence.

An eight-ball of cocaine, so called because it weighs 1/8 of an ounce, is about 3½ grams with a street price of around $150. In pharmaceutical literature we talk about the LD50 of a medication. That's the dose that is the lethal dose for 50 percent of the people taking it. Cocaine has an LD50 of about 1.2 grams for an average sized adult.

Cocaine addicts boast about how much cocaine they can snort, but it's a very capricious drug. When I was in training as an ear, nose, and throat resident we used cocaine regularly in nasal surgery. We'd coat a cotton-tipped applicator with pure cocaine flakes and insert it at strategic parts of the nose. It gave great anesthesia and was a potent vasoconstrictor (makes blood vessels constrict so they don't bleed).

I was learning about this from one of my attending physicians, Dr. Tom Johnson. Tom was preparing to do some nasal surgery on a patient under local cocaine anesthesia. The first thing he did was to get an IV started.

"Why the IV?" I asked. "It's just a quick local procedure."

He started to insert the cocaine applicators. "Just watch out if they get a headache," he said.

On cue, the patient said, "God, I've got a splitting headache starting right now."

Without missing a beat, Tom pulled the applicators and injected a bolus of Valium into the IV tubing. Less than five seconds later, the patient started a full-blown seizure right in front of my startled eyes.

"That's why the IV," he said. "Cocaine gives you a few seconds warning before the seizure starts. You can never tell who's going to have this kind of reaction, even if they've had cocaine anesthesia before."

I was a believer and still am. I don't know how many patients I've treated for cocaine-induced seizures who've later told me they'd been using for years without any problem. It can happen at any time and in any dose. So if you needed another reason not to do drugs...

X-ray machines, metal detectors, body searches and drug-sniffing dogs are all employed to cut down on contraband in penal institutions, but they only catch a small proportion of the drug trade. Most prisoners will tell you that they can get pretty much anything they want just as easily in jails or prison as on the outside.

In jail tools and instruments can't be allowed to go missing. It's too easy for them to resurface as weapons. Each one is accounted for by signing them out to the responsible person and counting each one on a daily basis.

The dentist has an instrument we're all familiar with called an explorer. It's that long pointy thing he uses to poke at your teeth looking for cavities. While some are reusable, ours were disposable. No matter, they still had to be counted. One day the count was one short. That's bad.

The missing instrument, 6½ inches of cold steel with a sharp point and knurled handle, along with a steel-shafted mirror that's also part of the set, was nowhere to be found. The dentist and dental assistant scoured the supply cabinet looking for an explorer that might have fallen into a dark corner somewhere. Nothing. They went through all the trash for the day. Nada. Security got involved at this point and the entire medical suite was turned upside down. Zip. Someone had made off with the instruments.

The facility was locked down, meaning all inmates were confined to their cells. Security started through a list of all the patients who had been in medical or dental that day. The deputies coming off shift were turned around and pressed into service. Evening light had faded and nobody was happy.

Midnight came and went with no results. All activity in the medical clinic was reviewed again. Who was there? When? All the trash in medical was searched again. The night passed into morning.

The dental assistant said the only thing that had happened was that maintenance had come by the clinic to fix a sticky drawer #2 on their console. The missing instruments weren't in that drawer. They were kept in drawer #6.

Grasping at straws, Lieutenant Tripp, the head of security in medical, rounded up the maintenance guy, Diego. He held up the instrument package.

"Hey, Diego, when you were in dental yesterday did you see one of their instrument sets that looked like this?"

It's hard to tell when Hispanics turn pale, but Diego tried. "Uh, yeah. I think I might have picked one up." He opened his rolling cart and produced the mirror and the explorer. "These the ones?"

"How did they end up in your cart?"

"Well, I saw them and thought they'd be cool to use, you know, like picking locks and stuff. Hell, they just throw 'em away."

"You were working on drawer #2. These are kept in #6."

"Naw, they must have misplaced it in #2."

"You weren't looking in the other drawers?"

"No way. I wouldn't do that. Anyway they had a bunch of 'em. I didn't figure they'd miss just one."

"They did."

"No shit, man. Sorry."

It was a tossup whether to kill Diego on the spot or hug him because the instruments were found. The lockdown and search cost about $5,000 in overtime and a lot more than that in worry. In the end, Diego got some serious re-education in the importance of tool control.

After the dust settled, the jail staff and the prisoners both expressed their relief to the dentist and his assistant that the instruments were found. They knew the penalties for letting tools go missing and were glad to see the dental folks exonerated.

I have to be careful in what's allowed in medical too. It might seem callous to deny a crutch, cane, or brace for an injured limb. These easily become weapons either in their native state or by modification.

If a patient with a painful knee used his cane to attack someone in the past, he doesn't get another one. Period. End of story. If a patient comes back from surgery with a cast or brace containing reinforcing metal rods, he doesn't get back in general population until it's healed and the offending object is gone.

If he has a brace with metal hinges or rods, the brace comes off if possible and a soft brace substituted. Just a month ago in one of the Colorado prisons, a reinforced knee brace slipped through. It ended up as four sharpened shivs, fortunately discovered before they could be used.

Twenty-Two

On ICE

The U.S Immigration and Customs Enforcement (ICE) is the investigative arm of the U.S. Department of Homeland Security with an annual budget of nearly $6 billion (with a B). What this means is ICE is big, numbering more than 20,000 employees all over the world.

Part of their job is running down illegal aliens, called removable aliens in government-speak, and shooing them back to their countries of origin. In 2012 they managed nearly two million aliens in various stages of immigration removal proceedings. They deported over 366,000 aliens, 191,000 of which had a criminal background.

While they're being cranked through the government machinery they have to stay somewhere. Every day ICE processes more than 1,300 aliens into detention centers. That's where CJC and similar facilities come in.

The illegals are known at CJC as ICE detainees. According to government regulations, they have to have a health screening within twelve hours of hitting the door and have a complete workup with physical and dental exams within two weeks.

They see the dentist and mental health providers and get shipped out to the emergency room as needed just like our home-grown felons. If you're going to get arrested as an illegal alien, the U.S. is your best choice.

The ICE detainees usually speak Spanish as their primary language since most hail from Mexico or Central America. CJC used to have an interpreter on call, but getting one in the right place at the right time was costly and a general headache. Fortunately I lived in south Florida for a few years before coming to Colorado. You *have* to speak Spanish there or be isolated from half the population. I brushed up with some Pimsleur Spanish lessons and did my own interviewing.

It was gratifying to see a frightened, beaten-down detainee come for an appointment and brighten immediately when I greeted him and started through the health questions in Spanish. Many were so relieved that the doctor spoke their language that they'd launch into a barrage of street Spanish that totally left me in the dust. *"Mas despacio, por favor."* More slowly, please.

Many had never seen a physician, and their health status varied all over the map. The average stay before they're shipped out is twenty-seven days, the same length as most of our other residents. That didn't give me much time to reverse a lifetime of neglect.

Not surprisingly they walked in with the same medical issues as anyone else: high blood pressure, seizures, diabetes, heart disease, and high cholesterol. Many were in varying stages of malnutrition and drug addiction.

Colorado is kind of a crossroads for illegal aliens making their way up from the border. It's not a bad choice. Just taking into account K-12 education, public health costs and costs of incarcerating illegals who are criminals, it costs Colorado over a billion dollars a year or about $600 for each native-born household in the state. In Colorado illegal aliens can get a driver's license and go to college with in-state tuition. Many come looking for a better life, but sizable portions are criminals with gang ties.

The federal government forbids businesses to hire undocumented aliens, but they don't mind doing it themselves. Last year, at least 60,000 immigrants worked in the federal government's network of detention centers—more than worked for any single employer in the country.

These guys don't get the $8 an hour that is Colorado's minimum wage. The numbers are slippery, but ICE detainees work for about thirteen cents an hour and many aren't paid at all. That's a terrific bargain if you're an employer, like CJC, who doesn't have to hire outside contractors to do the work. If the prisoners use the money to buy something at the commissary, well, it's a company store.

If this sounds suspiciously like slavery, you're not far off. But slavery is illegal isn't it? At the end of the Civil War, the 13th Amendment abolished slavery … almost.

Included in the amendment was an item called the punishment clause. It says that slavery and involuntary servitude remain lawful "as a punishment for crime whereof the party shall have been duly convicted."

The rationale for this exception harks back to the Northwest Ordinance of 1787, the legislation that created the Northwest Territory in the young United States. At the time, hard work was believed to be essential to a prisoner's moral rehabilitation. Slavery, under that philosophy, was for the prisoner's own good.

In the 20th century, the Supreme Court did away with actual slavery, but the language is unchanged in the 13th Amendment to this day. This leaves enough wiggle room to put prisoners to work for little or no pay.

This is not to say that illegals are all innocent victims.

Going to jail is the first step in going to prison, which is the first step in recruiting gang members. Street gangs have gone international. Gangs that had their origins in cities like Los Angeles have spawned prison branches that spill into Latin America.

Gangs in L.A., for instance, led to the rise of gangs in Guatemala such as the ultra-violent Mara Salvatrucha 13, MS-13. A common cycle would be for a Guatemalan gang member to slip into the United States. He then commits a crime that earns him a couple of years in jail or prison. During his stay he recruits fellow inmates into the gang, increasing their power and income.

When he is released and deported back to Guatemala, the cycle repeats again, maybe in New Mexico next time. The prisons in Guatemala are training grounds for these recruiters, just as these men train recruiters in American prisons and jails.

Some of the illegals are just free-loaders. A recent incident in Boulder caught my eye in this regard. A man was caught in a flash flood. His car rolled upside down in the rushing water, and it took about two hours for first responders and divers to extract him.

You might expect someone in that position to be grateful, but instead he sued his rescuers because they didn't get him out fast enough. He claimed he had shoulder pain and demanded a half million bucks. It turned out that he was an illegal alien and "just wanted some money to pay my bills."

I'm not saying this kind of behavior is the exclusive province of illegals. We've got plenty of home-grown jerks that do the same or worse. The real problem in these cases is that there are lawyers willing to file these bogus complaints in the first place. End of rant.

Taking care of the illegals is a tough business. If I identify a significant medical problem in an ICE detainee, I first educate the patient about what it is and why he should care about it. Then what to do?

For instance, I can start him on blood pressure medication, but it's likely he won't be at CJC long enough for me to monitor the results and make sure he's on the correct medicine at the correct dose.

My prescription lasts until he gets discharged or deported. Then he's got to find his own doctor to carry on the treatment. Lots of times that isn't going to happen. When he leaves he probably won't be able to get the same medication, or perhaps any medicine at all. He's got to feed his family. Hypertension medication and doctor visits are on the luxury list.

The illegals who weren't in gangs were polite and agreeable, almost to the point of invisibility. They'd smile and nod, agreeing with whatever I said, accept the medicine and then vanish. If I had a chance to see them at a subsequent clinic, I'd often find that they hadn't taken the medicine I'd prescribed.

When I asked the reason, they'd just smile and shrug. They were very fatalistic about their lots in life, and while they might have thought I was a nice guy, they also had made up their minds that whatever I did wasn't going to make any difference.

They were probably right, but occasionally a light would go on. Someone would get excited that something could be done to stop the seizures or tack twenty years onto his life by controlling his hypertension or cholesterol. They might have a doctor back home who'd said the same thing, but now, for some reason, they understood and believed. Those are the times I thought the day had been worthwhile.

ICE detainees are in a special limbo legal class. They are housed in county jails on the basis of ICE detainer holds. In essence, it's a request by ICE for the local sheriff to hold a person in jail until they determine his immigration status.

This takes time, and frequently people are held in jail long after they would be released on other charges. For example, someone might be arrested for a minor traffic violation. If he is unable to provide identification and there is a suspicion that he might be an illegal alien, the jail may hold him until ICE can determine his status.

To incarcerate someone in Colorado, the jail is supposed to have a warrant, a document approved by a judge. The ICE request is just that, a request to jail someone without a warrant. Other states have determined this is illegal, and it certainly seems to be.

ICE in Colorado has come up with a special form, an I-200, that supposedly takes the place of a warrant, but it's still not approved by a judge. Several Colorado jails have already said they won't honor these anymore, but El Paso County is still "studying the matter."

It seems the reason to keep "studying the matter" is the income derived from housing ICE detainees. It's worthwhile to know if a person is an illegal alien or not, but jailing people for an indefinite period without a warrant while the feds review his credentials seems pretty creepy to me. Wasn't that how the Germans did it? Just sayin'…

TWENTY-THREE

VERBAL AIKIDO

What comes through the door in medical isn't all high blood pressure and seizures. I see problems as diverse as the clientele I serve.

Lucille, a chronic shoplifter, plunked her ample derriere on my exam table. "I want every STD test you got," she said. "I just found out my husband's a whore." And according to the testing I did, she was right.

Close behind, Elmore, a skinny smash-and-grab burglar, demanded, "I want an STD."

"You do?"

"Damn right. Everybody on my floor's got an STD, and I want one too."

"A question first," I said. "Do you know what an STD is?"

"Course I do. I ain't stupid. You gonna give me one or not? I know my rights."

"Giving out STDs isn't in my line," I said. "Mostly people get them elsewhere and then come to me afterwards."

"Like you got a collection?" he huffed.

"I could give you some numbers where you could pick up STDs when you get out."

"Do I look like I got the money to go buy my own STD?"

Well, Elmore had me there. Rather than engage in a fruitless attempt at education, I gave him his STD. Sort of. Just let it drop.

While maybe not Einsteins, lots of my patients were smart enough. However, a significant proportion just didn't make the grade. Marat Novotny, a Russian ex-pat with a seizure disorder, seemed typical of the breed. He sat poised on the edge of the exam table, hands folded precisely in his lap, radiating attention.

"Mr. Novotny, when was the last time you had a seizure?"

"I don't know, Doctor."

"It says on your intake form that you have seizures. Is that right?"

"That's what they tell me."

"Who tells you?"

"People tell me." He smiled, anxious to please. Eager and impenetrable.

"What people? Deputies at the jail?"

He shook his head. "I don't know who they were. My English…"

"When was the last time they told you that you had a seizure?"

"I'm not sure. I was having a seizure I think, so I don't remember so good."

"This year?"

"Might be. I'm not so good with dates."

"Do you take medicine for seizures?"

Marat brightened. "I take a green pill and a yellow one."

"They're for seizures?"

"Nobody told me what they were for. They might be for seizures." He hesitated and frowned. "Maybe not."

About now the only thing I'm sure of is I'm going to need a drink pretty soon.

Robbie Storms, a homeless recluse, slouched mute on my exam table. Shrugs and nods met my initial questions. Every few minutes I'd hear a sort of slurping sound like he might have severe nasal congestion.

"Can you tell me if you have any heart problems?" I asked.

Shrug.

"You sound like you're having some breathing problems," I offered hopefully.

Robbie kind of screwed up his mouth and gave a so-so nod.

Giving up on questioning, I decided to proceed to the physical exam. His nose didn't look all that congested. There was a pungent odor, but that wasn't particularly unusual for my patients.

"Let's have a look in your throat," I offered, poised with my light and tongue depressor. Robbie just shook his head.

"It's okay. I won't choke you. Just open up." He pursed his lips and shook even more definitively.

I switched into command mode. "Just a quick look, Mr. Storms. I've really got to." The deputy in the hall edged closer, anticipating possible trouble. Robbie looked over his shoulder at the deputy and back to me. He was almost in tears.

"Okay," he mumbled and spread his lips apart with his fingers. The stench nearly knocked me back. I saw a jumble of wires and gums swollen with pus.

"What the hell happened to you?" I said involuntarily. I realized where the slurping sound originated.

Long story short, Robbie had fractured his jaw in a fight eleven years ago during a previous incarceration. He was taken to an oral surgeon who wired the upper and lower jaws together so the fracture could heal. Robbie was so afraid of the pain he might have taking the wires off that he just left them on. For eleven years.

The wires had cut through the gums and the bases of the teeth leading to a chronic draining infection in every tooth left in his mouth. I gave Robbie a pat on the back and escorted him around the corner to Mike, my dentist buddy.

"Hey, Mike, you busy?"

"Not too bad. Kind of slow today," he said.

"I can fix that."

Methamphetamine addiction is a problem not only medically, but also for the dentist. "Meth mouth," the destruction of the teeth from amphetamine use, is common in our patients. I asked Mike how that worked. He's a frustrated professor and quickly warmed to the subject.

He explained that teeth enamel is a matrix of calcium and phosphorus. Anything in the mouth with an acid pH lower than 5.5 will literally dissolve the enamel. Meth smoke has a pH of 1. Since most meth smokers often center the pipe to smoke it, the thinner-enameled front teeth get the brunt of it.

The erosion starts with a little black hole at the gum line and just gets worse and worse as the enamel erodes away. Bruxism and mouth dryness caused by the drug accelerate the fracture and decay.

Because meth mouth is such a bear to treat, Mike often ends up extracting multiple unsalvageable teeth in the process. Even anesthesia is a problem as the infection interferes with local anesthetics.

"What do you do then?" I asked.

"Well, if Septocaine and Lidocaine aren't working, there's always Hammercaine."

"Hammercaine? Oh..." So if you needed another reason to say no to drugs...

I asked Mike about the types of patients he saw with dental problems. His answer, only partially tongue-in-cheek, was he subtracted ten IQ points for every missing front tooth. Probably not a bad rule of thumb.

Our dental assistant is Carmelita, a fiery half-German, half-Cherokee lady with a laugh like a rhinoceros. Actually, I'm not sure what a laughing rhinoceros sounds like, but you get the idea. It's forceful.

Carmelita's strategy in dealing with nervous inmates is to have a great offense. In between patient's she'll go out in the waiting room filled with felons, plunk herself down in a chair and have a gab session. When they come back to the dental chair, she's a combination of Mother Teresa and Jim Carrey.

Carmelita is an ambassador for the dental department. She owns seventy pair of sneakers to color-coordinate with her wardrobe of scrubs. Color matching goes to her earrings and even her watches. I asked her why she went to so much trouble to come work at the jail.

"It's a matter of respect," she said. "If I take the time to iron my scrubs and dress with care, it reflects the care that people will receive when they come to see us in dental. We're scrutinized by our patients, and if they see someone who dresses carelessly, it communicates that they're going to get shoddy care. I want to give them more than they expect."

She counsels her patients, holds hands, whispers comforting reassurance, and tells jokes. She has an arsenal of inspirational quotations and posters. On their birthdays she lets them pick the music she plays in the clinic. I don't hear screams from the dental room, I hear maniacal laughter.

After the dentist administers the anesthetic for a procedure, Carmelita swings into action with jokes, inspiration, and life lessons that keep the patient busy, distracted, and anxiety-free for fifteen minutes while the drug takes effect. She's had more than one patient say that he'd pay the $8 fee just to come and talk with her for twenty minutes.

Not everyone takes to dental treatment. Some get downright nasty, but Carmelita's ready. A recent visitor made a *sotto voce* comment that sounded a lot like the c-word. Carmelita didn't miss a beat. "C-U-N-T? You mean like 'See You Next Tuesday?' I don't work on Tuesdays, so it'll have to be 'See You Next Wednesday.'" She can pull this off without cracking a smile while looking them straight in the eye. Nobody ever comes back for a second helping.

Carmelita is an attractive woman in a largely male environment. It's common for her to garner looks from the inmates, but when it turns to leers she takes the bull by the horns.

She walks up to the leerer and demands," Do I remind you of someone?" Backpedaling quickly under Carmelita's laser glare, he stammers, "Uh, no ma'am. No. I apologize for, uh, anything." She'll give a curt nod of acknowledgement and leave the miscreant in a pool of sweat.

Since Carmelita is the point woman for dental patients, I asked if she had any procedures in place for dealing with an unruly client. She smiled and escorted me back to her instrument cabinet.

"This is a luxator," she said, holding up a wicked-looking 6" pointy thing with a knurled handle. "This is an elevator," holding up an equally lethal other-pointy thing.

"Can you imagine," she continued, casually palming the luxator, "what distress this would cause if jabbed into your temple? The deputy said there wouldn't be an investigation." Oookayyy…

I asked Mike, the dentist, if he'd ever encountered a tense situation while seeing jail patients. He thought for a minute and then said, "Well, there was the time when the lights went out.

"I was seeing a guy from segregation, one of the bad-asses. I had a Minnesota retractor in his cheek and a high-speed drill revved up in my other hand. Carmelita was down the hall getting some suture when the power went out."

I should mention that the dental clinic, like every other room in medical, has no windows, and when the power goes off it's really, really dark. To make things worse, it's around the corner and down the hall from the rest of medical with no deputies standing outside.

"So I'm sitting there with the drill whining away about an inch from this guy's face and the retractor in his cheek. There's a whole tray of instruments including scalpels and such within the inmate's reach. He knows that, and I know that, and he knows that I know that."

"So?" I asked.

"I cranked the retractor over as far as I could. At least I knew where his head was. I had the drill, and I was listening for any rattle of the instrument tray."

"And? And?"

"And the lights came back on. Everybody was happy, but they were off long enough for both of us to run through a lot of scenarios."

Aikido is a martial art centered on disrupting your opponent's balance. You never oppose your partner's energy, but simply redirect it. By not opposing your opponent's strength, you give him nothing to push against.

It's very dancelike and meditative unless you happen to be the opponent somersaulting onto your backside.

In my younger, more nimble days I got one of my three black belts in aikido. While it's a handy physical skill to have in a prison, verbal aikido is every bit as useful.

Jails are full of argumentative people. Like slime in swamps, it goes with the territory. And argumentative people like to—can you guess?—argue.

I never mind discussing reasons for my clinical decisions, but I don't like to argue about them. Once I've decided the best course to take, I'm pretty much done with hashing over pointless objections. If there's a real reason why I should or shouldn't do something, I've already taken some pains to discover it.

Most of the time my argumentative patients want to get something they don't need or shouldn't have, like a thicker mattress, more pain medications or a trip to the Bahamas. Unless I want to stir up an ulcer, it's best to avoid the aggravation that outright refusal generates. I do this with verbal aikido.

Take my recent encounter with Kevin Ulrich, a 285-pound ball of meanness. Kevin wanted some narcotics for his chronic back pain. I'd already determined that his back pain was muscular in origin secondary to his weightlifting hobby. I've talked to him about stretching and other physical therapy that he could do himself, but he's focused on a pharmaceutical solution.

"You gotta give me something stronger for this pain. That ibuprofen and Tylenol aren't doing anything for it. I need Vicodin or Percocet. That's what my doctor gave me before I came here."

Now it would be easy and direct to just say no. What I can count on if I take this route is an argument about how severe his pain is versus my intransigence in not giving him stronger pain medications. He's the good guy; I'm the bad guy.

What I can also count on is he won't give up his quest. If I refuse his request outright, I'll get more kites on the same subject, and grievances about deliberate indifference will flow to administration. Aggravation all around. So I take another tack.

"Hmm. How long has this been going on?" Notice I didn't say no or deny his complaint of pain. Just gathering information. Trying to help. Can't object to that, can he?

"Ever since that car wreck in 2005. Been screwed up ever since."

"So you saw a doctor who gave you Percocet?" The noose is starting to tighten.

"Yeah, he always gave me Percocets."

"Great," I say. "I'll get his information so we can follow his treatment plan. What's his name? He's in Denver?" See? I'm on Kevin's side, trying to get the best care for him. Nothing to push against here.

"I don't remember his name. He's at that big hospital downtown." Now I know he's lying about having a regular doctor. He's either been getting his pills from ER visits or from his buddies on the street. But I don't call him on it. No need.

"Big hospital downtown? Maybe Swedish?"

"Yeah, I think that's it."

"Terrific. I'll send a request for information to Swedish, and we'll get you on the right medicines." Notice I didn't say what the right medicines were. He's already taking them. I know there's no doctor at Swedish Hospital, and I'm not going to get an answer to my request for information, but Kevin's lied his way into a box. Not my fault. I'm still on his side, just trying to solve the problem. Time to narrow the field a little.

"You know CJC doesn't allow any narcotics in the building, so we'll have to work around that as best we can." Kevin knows this already, but I'm pointing it out not as something I just thought up, but rather as a policy I couldn't change even if I wanted to. You'll notice it's something *we* work on, not just me. Not my fault. I'm on his side.

"At least I need an increase in the ibuprofen or Tylenol."

"I'm worried that the ibuprofen will make your acid reflux worse. It's famous for doing that. The Tylenol's a problem because of being toxic to your liver. I'm trying to not cut the doses you're taking now. I'm concerned they might be too much to use long-term. What do you think?"

Kevin realizes he's not going to get the narcotics he wants, and now I've raised the prospect of decreasing the medicines he already has access to. Game over.

"No. I think they're okay. Let's keep them going for a while. I'll let you know if my stomach acts up."

Kevin leaves the clinic with relief, having held on to his OTC medicines. He's not going to kite again over the same issue because he knows I might cut them back due to concerns for his health. Best to let sleeping dogs lie.

Throughout all this exchange I never said no to his request or cast doubt on his veracity. We've worked together on a problem instead of arguing about it. He may not be thrilled with the result, but at least it works, and he can continue with a rational therapy.

Is this manipulative? You bet it is. Is it disrespectful? I don't think so. I'm trying to get Kevin to buy into what I think is the best therapy for him. Arguing isn't going to do it. Verbal aikido may take a little longer than just saying no, but creating a win-win situation leaves everyone with lower blood pressure, including me.

TWENTY-FOUR

ROMANCE

One of the drawbacks of being in jail is the limited opportunity for dating. A possible remedy reportedly originated in the California prison system. Inmates began "sagging," that is, wearing their pants low enough to display a significant swatch of underwear or worse. Justin Bieber is a proponent of sagging, which should be reason enough for others to avoid the practice.

The California prisoners supposedly adopted this dress to signal that they were "available" or that they were "already taken." Probably it came about because, like all occupants of jails and prisons, they didn't have belts.

Women being in short supply in jail, some male inmates resort to being "gay for the stay." Since being gay would seem to be the antithesis for successful survival in a testosterone-fueled prison setting, how can men have homosexual relationships and yet avoid the stigma of being regarded as homosexual?

There are a couple of requirements for carrying this off. First, the homosexual acts must represent only a situational reaction to the deprivation of heterosexual relations. If these men could have their choice, they'd pick a woman. It's like getting away with eating steak if you're a vegetarian. All you have to do is convince your peers that you'd rather have broccoli.

Just as important, the behavior must have a complete absence of emotion or feminine trappings. If a man demonstrates a convincing façade of toughness and "manliness," he can avoid being labeled as "weak" or "queer." You can see how this precludes warm, fuzzy homosexual relationships.

The few studies that address this issue divide participants into the "voluntary aggressors" and the "involuntary recruits." The recruits tend to be among the weakest and youngest inmates, usually approached within a couple of days of their admission.

The voluntary aggressors tend to be older, stronger, and more ingrained in the jail or prison hierarchy. Frequently they are gang members.

Like the vegetarians forced by hunger to eat a steak, they never saw themselves as homosexual despite participating in homosexual acts. Aggression, power, and dominance were the main ingredients in their activities. Upon release they tended to resume heterosexual relationships, albeit with a continued element of the violence and dominance they experienced in confinement.

They knew the person they were having sexual relations with was a male, but they didn't view him as such. They considered him a "substitute" for a female. They saw themselves performing as straight people on another who was "queer."

Bryce McBride weighed in at close to 300 pounds and had hair growing out of every opening in his jump suit. Though quite fat, McBride appeared in pretty good shape and seemed an imposing 100 percent manly presence on my suddenly tiny exam table.

"Can I pull this curtain, Doc?" he said.

"Sure. What's up?"

"I got this…you know."

"Not really."

"You know, down there," he said, pointing to his crotch.

"Ah. Let's take a look."

He glanced back at the curtain and dutifully dropped his drawers.

"You've got herpes," I said. "Is this the first time?"

He reddened. "Herpes! I got herpes? You sure?"

"That's what it is. Hurt?"

"Like a mother," he sputtered.

"We'll get you on some medication for it. If this is the first time, it may cure it."

"That little bastard!" he roared.

The deputy drew back the edge of the curtain. "You okay, Doc?"

"We're good," I said. "Just a little surprise."

McBride, a white supremacist gang member and possibly one of the leaders, by no means fit the stereotype of a gay man. The ethos of the gang prohibited homosexuality, yet he had obviously jumped the fence. He wasn't in protective custody, so he apparently was doing it with the tacit approval of the gang or was lucky enough to hide it.

Inmates are more likely to be raped if they've been convicted of a sexual offense, especially against a juvenile. Anyone with feminine characteristics or an attitude of weakness is prime game. If they succumb, they are irrevocably marked as "punks" or "damaged goods," much like a woman who has been the victim of rape.

Punks are on the lowest rung of the ladder. Although they may enjoy some measure of protection early on, they are slaves to be used, traded away in card games, or sold for cigarettes. Advice within the prison community to potential victims is to fight like hell rather than give in. The pain of a beating will be less than the pain of what follows submission. At least the potential recruit gains some respect, and respect is the currency of the incarcerated.

Recruits may have thought they had no alternative but to submit, that this was the only path to survival, very much like the method of survival in concentration camps. One recruit said in an interview, "You get used to anything. You got to live. And I suppose getting used to it, you get to like it. Liking it is your way of getting used to it."

Although heterosexual before being incarcerated, recruits often maintain a homosexual lifestyle after release. It seems that they came to see themselves as others saw them.

The deputies brought Jeffrey Rachel to the medical clinic suffering from multiple bruises around the throat and arms. A slight, blonde man of twenty years, his eyes darted nervously from side to side continuously as if expecting a hidden attack at any moment. He sat in my exam room, hands clasped in his lap and shoulders hunched.

"What happened, Mr. Rachel?" I asked.

"I fell."

"Anybody help you fall?"

"No. I slipped in the bathroom."

"I see. You mind if I take a look?"

He shrugged. I did an exam that showed abrasions on the neck, arms, and legs compatible with being held down.

"Somebody try to assault you?"

"No. I..." Tears flowed down his cheeks.

"Just wait here a minute, okay?"

He turned his head away and nodded numbly.

I notified the shift commander that I suspected Rachel was a rape victim. It might have been a simple assault, but the markings suggested something more sinister. No fool, the shift commander was already in the clinic, believing this to be the case.

I referred Rachel on to one of the rape investigators, since this was likely a criminal matter now. For the rest of his stay at CJC, Rachel was housed in medical under protective custody. If returned to general population, there was a good chance he would be attacked again.

In the last decade jails and prisons have adopted many proactive measures to curb homosexual relations. In 2003 Congress passed the Prison Rape Elimination Act (PREA) to study the problem and facilitate solutions. Every year I have training in PREA concepts and awareness, which boils down to "in prison there are no consensual sexual relations."

This recognizes that jails and prisons are coercive environments—one person or group having power over another. Gangs run the sex trade through intimidation. Jail staff has obvious power over the inmates. American criminals have advantages over ICE detainees who suffer a cultural and language deficit. Big guys can dominate little guys. Men can generally dominate women (unless you're my wife).

This led to a zero tolerance policy for sex of any kind in a jail or prison setting. Even though the participation may have been voluntary on both sides, the assumption is that somebody forced somebody else to have sex.

If you get caught having sex with someone, you're guilty of rape. Period. It's one of those policies that may not be 100 percent correct, but it saves a lot of finger pointing and puts the aggressors on notice that they'll be punished regardless of the story they come up with.

Unless something is life-threatening, I didn't examine supposed rape victims. They were seen by a PREA-trained practitioner familiar with forensics, as well as by the deputies tasked with the investigation.

Relationships aren't just with other inmates. Civilians get tangled up with prisoners on a regular basis. Back in my home state of Indiana, a female senior judge who defended a 26-year-old male inmate when practicing as his attorney was barred from the jail after video monitors showed her engaging in "excessive fondling" of her former client. It turned out they had been carrying on an affair for a couple of years.

Visitation rules allowed a "brief hug and kiss," but they found this too limiting and retired to a side room for greater exploration. The judge thought this was beyond the range of the cameras, but was busted for the escapade.

In Fort Worth Wesley Miller was convicted of the murder of an 18-year-old cheerleader, becoming the first killer committed under Texas' Sexually Violent Predator Program. After his release he was required to live at the jail and was returned to formal custody several times for refusing to participate in sex-offender counseling and for additional sexual offenses.

None of this made a difference to the 21-year-old female jailer who decided that Miller was a great catch and carried on an affair with him at the Cold Springs Jail. You just have to wonder.

CJC contracts food services with an outside company. They supervise the food handling and preparation with trustee inmates providing the labor. One of their supervisors was walked out of the jail after being busted for giving and receiving oral sex with his inmate crew. No, I do not want to know what's in the lasagna.

Inmates attach themselves to civilians like lampreys on a lake trout. In their disadvantaged position they're looking for not only emotional support but also all things financial. This can get ugly, but my favorite story is about the flip side where the civilian turned the tables.

Abhelhafid Rahmani (I am not making this up), a native of Morocco, is currently serving two life prison sentences in Florida for murdering his first wife and her husband. Undeterred by this unfortunate glitch in marital relations, Casilda Sanchez-Fernandez, a paralegal, struck up a jailhouse romance with Rahmani and eventually married him at the state prison.

Romance bloomed. Sanchez-Fernandez ponied up $20,000 for Rahmani's legal expenses plus $300 a month for jail spending money. She bought him new teeth and glasses and even paid $7,000 for his niece to go to college. Sanchez-Fernandez began to notice that this relationship was all give and no get. Things started to go south.

Rahmani wanted to appeal his murder convictions. Sanchez-Fernandez wanted out of this one-sided paper marriage. Knowing he had a sucker on the line, he refused to sign the divorce papers.

Rahmani needed his trial transcript and case paperwork to file along with his appeal. Sanchez-Fernandez had the papers at home. Heh heh heh…

Unless Rahmani signed divorce papers, Sanchez-Fernandez threatened to burn the papers. She even wrote and told him, "You can kiss them good-bye."

He appealed to the judge, but got no relief. Eventually he signed the divorce papers and the judge ordered his now-ex-wife to give back his paperwork. She did. After the appeals deadline had passed.

"Revenge is sweet and not fattening."

—Alfred Hitchcock

Prison pen pals are fertile ground for catastrophe. Prisoners need love too, but it's a great arena for scams. Here are a few caveats before you pick up your pen:

Find out who you're dealing with. People are often in jail because they are honesty-impaired. Do a little research and find out why they're in jail in the first place. An inmate might (surprise!) not be telling the truth about this offense or previous ones. Read the trial records. Is this a guy you want to deal with? Really?

Remember, this is a prisoner you're dealing with. They are often skilled in deception and manipulation. They'll tell you whatever they think you need to hear, probing for your weaknesses to get their hooks in.

Be careful revealing personal details, especially finances. Prisoners usually don't have much in the way of cash, and they'd love to have you send some of yours. Don't start with money and gifts.

Be stingy with personal information. Remember, you may want to separate yourself from this guy in the future. Getting a PO box to avoid giving a home address is a good idea. Keep information about your kids and relatives and where you work private.

Someday this guy is going to be released, and your nice little home looks a lot better than the halfway house or the street. If your prisoner pen pal tries to align his future with yours, watch out. Make sure he knows that is not an option.

Remember that as much as your prison pen pal loves you, he probably loves others just as much or more. He's got nothing but time, and he can't put all his eggs in one basket. The heart-shrouded letter he sends to you likely has many duplicates going out at the same time. Keep in mind that you might be only one of several correspondents.

Don't, don't, *don't* send sexy pictures. Just don't. Even if they got by the jail's censors, they're passed around and used as currency for cigarettes or other items. How many boyfriends do you want?

On a similar note, don't talk sex on the phone or in writing. The censors are watching and listening. 'Nuff said.

With all these cautions, helping someone with emotional support can be very gratifying. You can be supportive without enabling their situation. Strive to make them stronger and more self-sufficient with your encouragement, but don't be a crutch or a shield from the realities they need to face.

TWENTY-FIVE

FAQ

One question that always comes up in discussions of correctional medicine is whether prisoners receive medical care comparable in quality to the rest of the population. By law prisoners have to receive medical care the same as the "community standard of care," so the answer is a qualified yes.

By qualified I mean cheap. Anyone with a TV set is subjected to advertisements for the latest and greatest drug. Latest and greatest doesn't necessarily mean better. Take someone with elevated cholesterol. Medications that have been around forever and are available as generic brands are almost always cheaper than the patent-protected newcomers.

How much cheaper? Pravastatin is a cholesterol-lowering drug we commonly use in correctional settings, but Crestor, a new drug that does essentially the same thing, is generally not available to us. Why? Without insurance to pay the bill, a thirty-day supply of Pravastatin costs about twelve bucks while Crestor runs over $200. We're on a budget, so our patients are too.

If an older, tried-and-true drug works as well as the new whiz-bang offerings, guess which ones are on our formulary. That's how it should be, and I seldom have a complaint about that. If I really need Crestor or whatever for a patient, I can usually pry it loose from the corporate bean-counters if I've got a good reason. As long as I've got something that works, I'm happy.

A problem that's just hit the medical community is the breakthrough success of new treatments for hepatitis C. Hep C, a viral liver disease that is transmitted blood-to-blood via tattoos and IV drugs, is endemic in jail and prison populations. We don't treat Hep C in jail because we don't have time to get the treatment done for most inmates, but I treated it routinely in prison settings.

The previous therapy wasn't cheap, and after a year of treatment we could only cure about 40 percent of people. Not great. Now hitting the market are new treatments that shorten the time to three months and cure 90 percent. We should be thrilled, right?

Depending on who you listen to, the new therapies will cost about $1,000 per pill. Let's see… A thousand bucks a pill times three months…you're looking at a hundred grand for medication cost per patient. There goes the budget.

Nobody's quite sure what to do about this yet. Fortunately for the corrections checkbook, the new treatments for Hep C aren't "community standard" yet, but they will be shortly. The shorter treatment times also puts pressure to offer treatment to jail detainees.

We have to remember that curing Hep C, while a worthwhile endeavor, doesn't confer any immunity to the disease. If we cure an inmate and he goes out and shoots up again or gets a new tattoo we're right back where we started, except for being $100,000 poorer.

Before we rush to judgment on this, consider the costs of treating the patients who progress to chronic liver failure. Not to put too fine a point on it, these folks often take a long, expensive time to check out. If you have a solution to this problem, write it on the back of a twenty-dollar bill and send it to me.

Isn't working in a jail depressing? I'd answer, "Compared to what?" Compared to touring the Côte-d'Or with a bevy of supermodels, yes. As a matter of fact, hell, yes. But compared to my former occupation as an ear surgeon, the answer is not as clear.

When I was in private practice, I was on the bottom of the food chain. Everybody got theirs, and I got what was left over. While that's great if there's a lot left over, it's the pits if there isn't. Every year I had to work harder to end up with less.

On top of that, I wasn't feeling much of the novelty and challenge that made medicine so exciting when I first started. When I found a new career in correctional medicine, things got fun again. I saw something new almost every day, and I could practice a wide scope of medicine instead of my little insular slice.

I was never a great administrator. I just expected people to do their jobs without me having to look over their shoulders and direct. Now I didn't have to do that anymore. I let someone else worry about schedules, personality clashes, hiring and firing. I could let someone else do the books, make payroll, and file the insurance claims. It was liberating. I could just practice medicine. At the end of the day, I could go home and forget about work.

I'll admit that my offices haven't been as upscale as they used to be, but then again, I don't have to pay for them. I don't have to concern myself with marketing my practice, and I can largely avoid the political infighting of the medical old boys' club. I can't avoid the political infighting of the sheriff's office and CHC's duplicity (more on that later), so I guess it's a draw on that point.

My patients are a big step down from what I was used to, but I get the sense that they need the help more. Although I don't see a lot of gratitude from the jail population, I really didn't get that much in private practice either. People seemed to feel that if they paid their bills, it wasn't important to also say thank you.

Note to patients: If your doctor does a good job, thank him. It doesn't cost you anything, and it will make his day.

So while there are downsides to correctional medicine, like getting killed, it's a pretty good gig. Next question.

Do you treat prisoners differently if they're in for something horrible? What about treating prisoners you don't like?

For the most part, I don't want to know what crime landed a prisoner in my clinic. If it's not pertinent to his medical care, it's really none of my business.

I do my best to avoid passing judgment on my patients. That's not my job. They're in prison or jail as punishment, and it's not my place to heap additional misery on their plates.

Having said that, if a prisoner did something off-the-wall horrible to get arrested, their personalities don't change on this side of the walls. If a person is an arrogant jerk on the outside, he'll likely be an arrogant jerk on the inside too.

I'll admit I don't do well with arrogant jerks, quite apart from rehashing their crimes. These people tend to get bare minimum services from me and a quick trip back out the clinic door. I'll take care of them, but no warm fuzzies.

If an inmate is rude and abusive during a clinic visit, they're out the door even faster. They can come back when they learn to behave. I had one patient, Elmo Givens, a sixty-something, white-haired bigot who had a grudge against most of North America. Elmo put in a kite to see me, but wouldn't elaborate about what the issue was.

"Hi, Mr. Givens. What brings you to the clinic today?"

"I been waiting out there for over an hour. I ain't gonna pay three bucks to wait on you all day."

"You've already paid your three bucks," I said. "What's the problem today?"

"You bloodsuckers are all the same. I ain't got money for this bullshit."

"You've got about thirty seconds to tell me what the problem is."

"The problem is you sons-of-bitches get off jacking me around. I—"

Despite my reddening face, I tried to keep my voice level. "Out."

"I'm not going anywhere. I came here to—"

"You came here to bitch. Come back when you can be civil." I motioned to the deputy, who had been inching closer during the exchange.

"You can't do this! I'm a ward of the state. I'm entitled to free medical care."

"Not free. Three bucks. Thanks for playing. Out." The deputy tightened his grip on Elmo's elbow and they left, Elmo trailing a stream of invective.

Elmo was a slow learner. On each of the next three visits he started in the same way, and each time was escorted, untreated, from the clinic. In the real world I could send Elmo a letter dismissing him as my patient, but neither of us had that luxury in the jail. I was the only game in town.

Just as Elmo couldn't get rid of me, I couldn't get rid of him either. I was the doctor for all the inmates, and if I didn't like somebody, too bad. Every time Elmo sent in a kite, I'd have to allow him in for another tirade. I was sorely tempted to pawn him off on the nurse practitioner, but she didn't deserve the grief either.

Aren't the doctors who go into corrections sort of bottom-of-the-barrel types? You know, people who couldn't make it in the real world?

In a word, no. Setting my own sterling qualifications aside, I've worked with a bunch of different medical providers (MDs, DOs, NPs, and PAs) in my nine years in corrections. While there are a few I wasn't too thrilled with, the vast majority were of equal caliber to my colleagues in private practice.

On the other hand, I've had several medical friends who gave correctional medicine a try and couldn't make it. Part of it was the inability to emotionally function in a prison environment with its unique rules and restrictions. It doesn't help if you're afraid of your patients.

For some, the breaking point came because they weren't able to do a million-dollar workup on every patient. While admirable from a theoretical standpoint, extensive workup of every problem isn't either necessary or cost-efficient.

The time is passing when doctors can blithely order costly testing just to bolster their clinical impressions or to ward off the possibility of malpractice suits. It's harder to rely on your own diagnostic abilities rather than ordering MRI scans "just to be sure." Some of my private practice friends couldn't make that leap to the limited resources of the correctional environment.

I don't say this to run them down. We need the specialists who will poke and prod into the dark corners and root out the obscure disorders. I rely on them when I've reached the limit of my abilities. But...

If the apocalypse hits tomorrow and all the laboratories and MRI scanners are reduced to rubble, I'd be very grateful to have a doctor who can think on his feet, make a good clinical diagnosis and initiate a reasonable treatment plan without all that ancillary help.

So am I a medical Luddite? Not at all. I love the technology, but I hate to see it being used as a substitute for thought. If I'm 90 percent sure that this patient has XYZ as a diagnosis, do I need to spend another five grand to cover the other 10 percent?

I probably do if the consequences of being wrong are catastrophic, but that's not usually the case. Most of my private patients were comfortable with me saying, "I'm 90 percent sure this is XYZ. We can start treatment and if it's no better in three or four weeks we can go looking for other possibilities." That's the way I run my clinic at the jail.

So are prison doctors inferior to those on the outside? No, they just operate in a different milieu. Correctional medicine places emphasis on good physical diagnosis skills and use of limited basic laboratory work, doing more with less.

It's not that we can't get the high-tech stuff. We just need a good reason for it, and that's as it should be. As long as overzealous administrators don't get in the way, we can practice the same standard of medicine as we did on the outside.

So why don't more doctors work in corrections? It certainly wasn't on the top of my list when I graduated from medical school. It wasn't on the list at all. In reality, it just never occurred to me. In the back of my mind I figured that since prisons were such grungy, horrible places, anybody who worked there must be of the same stripe.

It wasn't until I was burned out in private practice that I really started searching for alternatives. As I look back, I'm sorry I didn't make the change sooner. That seems to be a common thread with correctional physicians. It's a corner of medicine we sort of stumble upon by accident later in our careers.

So why did I choose to migrate to corrections instead of some more socially acceptable line of work? I really don't know. It was the first thing that really struck me as being a new and interesting way of supporting my family. I suppose if something else had come along at that vulnerable moment, I would have caromed off in another direction. If they'd needed a medical director for the Swedish bikini team…

How does working in the jail affect your home life? What does your wife think about you working in such a place?

At first my wife, Mollie, thought I was nuts for considering taking a job in corrections. Until I got established, I often thought the same thing. After I got the hang of working in jails and prisons, Mollie saw how much happier I was when I got home at night. I was doing something I was reasonably good at, and medicine as a profession was fun again. After putting up with my grousing about private practice, the change was thrilling for her.

I relieved some of her concerns about working in a prison when I brought her to family night at the supermax prison. This outreach by the warden to educate family members of prison staff about what the working environment was really like served to allay a lot of fears and misconceptions. Mollie commented about how neat and clean the place was.

By the time I took over the medical director's slot at the jail, Mollie wasn't too worried about me. She was a nurse before becoming an artist, so she concentrated on asking what interesting cases I'd seen that day. If I had some particularly notorious inmate, I might tell her about him, but she respected my preference to not investigate the reasons my patients ran afoul of the law.

An advantage of correctional medicine is the ability to leave work at work. I had to take phone calls from CJC when I wasn't on premises, but the issues were usually minor and quickly handled. I dealt with more serious issues by scheduling them in my clinic the next day. If needed, I could send an emergency out to the ER.

Compared to the stress of running my private practice, working in corrections was a walk in the park. I think the improved attitude I brought home had a positive effect on my marriage too. Mollie couldn't help but be affected by the negativity I'd developed in private practice, and its absence lifted a weight from both of us.

Twenty-six

The Corporate Culture

As the Medical Director of the El Paso County Criminal Justice Center (I just like to spell out the whole thing every once in a while. Seems impressive, doesn't it?) I am the master of all I survey…to a point. In truth I'm a cog in the corporate gears of my actual employer, Correctional Healthcare Corporation (CHC).

CHC is a giant amalgamation of eight separate correctional industry companies that all got glommed together in 2011. Based in a suburb of Denver, CHC contracts to provide healthcare services to about 250 facilities in twenty-seven states. This accounts for medical services to 70,000 inmates nationwide. Makes my domain of 1,500 patients look pretty puny.

Their website is filled with testimonials about how great it is to work for CHC, along with the obligatory pictures of smiling multiethnic people strangely tilted over at about a 15° angle. That may be for artistic purposes, or perhaps a nod to Colorado's mountainous terrain. Whatever.

I'm a fan of Clive Cussler's books featuring Dirk Pitt, his answer to Indiana Jones. Pitt tours the world saving the oceans and mankind from nefarious schemes while destroying millions of dollars of hardware. Great stuff.

I was surprised to see that CHC's president and CEO is also named Dirk. This wasn't mentioned in my orientation materials. It's not a common name. Could there possibly be a connection? His corporate picture doesn't resemble what I imagined Dirk Pitt might look like, but with Photoshop you never know. CHC's Dirk is kind of balding and is maybe carrying a few extra pounds, while Cussler's has a full head of hair and an Adonis physique. Naw, the name's probably just a coincidence.

Down the pecking order is the Chief Medical Officer, Dr. Raymond Herr. Ray supervises all the CHC medical personnel, including me. Wendy, my Health Services Administrator on site at CJC, is my boss too. The Sheriff, Terry Maketa, is also sort of my boss. When I signed on at CJC it was made plain to me that we were all here to keep the sheriff happy. Actually, I never was sure *who* my boss was, since everybody wanted to take a swing at it.

Medical services in jails and prisons can't just wing it. They have to be accredited by a boatload of oversight organizations with impressive initials. They perform audits of the most mind-numbing details you can imagine. Overall it's a good thing and keeps the care standards high. That doesn't mean the care is necessarily high, but at least the standards are.

Before I got recruited for CJC, the rumors going around were not favorable. I heard they were going to lose their accreditation due to a lot of inbred sloth and laziness. Whether this was true or not, I don't know, but it kept me from pursuing any inquiries about employment there.

When the new team of Wendy, the Health Services Administrator, and Denise, the Director of Nursing, came on board, things turned around with a vengeance. Remember, this is all rumor mill stuff as far as I was concerned.

In any case, the bad rumors stopped and the good rumors started. Then I got my invitation to come for an interview. Everyone, of course, loved me. I was on the team. I thought.

Practicing correctional medicine in a corporate environment is different from practicing in a state-run prison, and there are various ways you can be employed.

When I first started in corrections I was an employee of the State of Colorado. I got paid by the state and participated in the state retirement plan. The state covered my malpractice insurance. Simple.

Private prisons are for-profit facilities that contract with the state to take overflows of lower risk prisoners with less severe medical needs. This puts a layer of corporate concerns and politics between me and the place I'm actually working. Working at the jail was like working in a private prison.

While this might not sound like a big deal, the problem arises from working for two masters. In theory all of our goals should be congruent. We want to deliver the best medical care while keeping an eye on the bottom line. That's where our goals diverge.

Since the sheriff can't deliver medical care himself, even though he tried (more on that later), he hires it done. Right now CHC has the contract to furnish those medical services, and CHC hires me and others to do the actual delivering.

My goal is to deliver the best care I can. Period. I understand the economics involved and I'm not out to break the bank, but the financial considerations are secondary to delivering good care.

My employer, CHC, is in it for the money. Not that there's anything wrong with that, as Seinfeld would say. They have to abide by all sorts of federal and state rules for the standard of care they deliver, and that pushes them in the direction of quality that I favor.

Someone has to pay for this. That would be the sheriff's department via the contract they negotiated with CHC. The sheriff is concerned that at least adequate medical care goes on in the jail. They can't have prisoners dropping dead right and left. Someone is almost sure to notice.

So I have to keep CHC happy, and they have to keep the sheriff happy. I have to keep the sheriff happy too, because if momma ain't happy… Still, we're all on the same team, right?

Only up to a point. I reached that point when I insisted that interference by the sheriff and his minions in the operation of the medical clinic was unacceptable. Nobody was supposed to be practicing medicine at CJC except me and my staff.

CHC paid lip service to the principle, but balked at actually telling the sheriff to go arrest criminals and leave delivering medical care to actual medical personnel.

For those of you old enough to remember, Leo Gallagher was a comedian who toured the country with an act featuring his Sledge-O-Matic. He often made social commentaries, and one I particularly liked went, "If you don't confront ignorance and stupidity, ignorance and stupidity will think it's okay."

The sheriff apparently thought it was okay to play doctor, and CHC thought it was okay to let him. This led to the inevitable showdown.

Twenty-seven

Psycho Bitch

The wheels started to come off my relationship with the corporate client when the undersheriff, Paula Presley, decided she wanted to be a doctor. Apparently she was used to controlling the medical clinic during the tenure of my predecessor, Dr. Eloise.

At first there were requests that certain inmates get appointments or specific medications. I protested formally that these things were not the province of the sheriff's office, but the requests for specific medical management kept coming.

I took the issue to my CMO and got an email back stating that I was the doctor and he supported my objection 100 percent. Sort of. Pretty much. As long as I kept the corporate client happy.

Incidents kept piling up. Since I wasn't getting any relief via the chain of command, I jumped the queue and requested an audience with Presley. Denied.

The pot boiled over one evening with a call from the detox facility. The nurses noticed that one of their clients had some bleeding from her ear after trying to clean it with a wad of toilet paper. No pain. Bleeding had stopped. Nothing else.

I told the nurse that it was almost certainly a small ear canal laceration and not to worry about it that night. I'd take a look in the morning.

A few minutes later I got a call back. The nurse relayed that the undersheriff wanted the patient treated right now. I repeated that Presley wasn't a doctor, immediate treatment wasn't needed, and I'd see her in the morning.

The next call was from Wendy, my HSA. "What's going on with this patient they want to send to the hospital?"

I was getting tired of this. "There's nothing going on with this patient," I explained. "She's not in any distress and doesn't need urgent treatment or to go to a hospital. Remember, I was an ear specialist for over thirty years before I started in corrections. Trust me on this."

Fuming, I sat down to my getting-cold dinner again.

"You'd better go in there," said my wife, Mollie.

"What for? There's nothing that needs treating. It's just this woman who wants to play doctor."

"You'd better go in there," Mollie repeated.

"Bullshit," I replied. We sat. Like my dinner, I cooled off. "Okay, but it's a total waste of time." I got in the car and drove over to CJC. I was entering the parking lot when my cell phone rang. Wendy again.

"They're sending the ambulance for the patient right now. Presley's direct order."

"Direct order, eh? It would be nice if someone with some actual medical experience was calling the shots. Since I'm here, do you want me to take a look or just wait for the EMTs to rush her off to the emergency room?"

"You're there at CJC?"

"Wouldn't miss it. Not often I get in on such a big case."

The sound of rapid thinking hummed over the airwaves. "Why don't you take a look?"

"Might as well. Hope I don't get in the way of the emergency crew. Call you back."

I picked through my key ring and entered the detox unit. I didn't hear any screaming. Good sign. The nurse was filling out transfer papers to send the patient to the ER.

"Can I have a look at the patient with the emergency?"

"Mrs. Salton," she said. "Right over here."

The nurse gratefully led me to a gaunt middle-aged woman watching television. I introduced myself.

"I understand your ear's been bothering you."

She nodded. "Been kind of itching for a couple of days."

"Let me have a look." I produced my otoscope and peered into her ear canal. The only abnormality was a small abrasion where she'd scrubbed around with the toilet paper wad.

"You've got a small cut in your ear canal where you tried to itch it," I explained. "Don't try to clean it anymore. We'll get some drops to prevent any infection from getting started."

"That would be great," she said, one eye remaining on her television show. "Could it wait until tomorrow? I don't want to miss the ending."

"Tomorrow sounds good."

I dialed Wendy and relayed the events. "You still want her to go to the hospital?"

"Call you back," she said.

A few minutes later the phone rang as I was trudging to the car. "Presley couldn't believe that you'd come in at night."

"Full service," I deadpanned. "She was probably counting on me not coming in, so she could run her little emergency without interference." I noticed that I was becoming more sarcastic.

"She said that since you've examined her, the ambulance wouldn't be necessary."

"She trusts me to make the call on that? Sure she doesn't want to come in and check out the situation herself? Give me a second opinion?"

I could hear Wendy take a deep breath. "I think it's all good. See you tomorrow, Dr. Wright."

You'd think that after such a public humiliation, Presley would pull in her horns, maybe even offer an apology for being such a jerk, but it was not to be. First, a little background.

Suboxone is an opioid medication used primarily in the treatment of narcotic addiction. It's in a restricted class of medication that requires special training before a doctor can prescribe it or a nurse can administer it.

We have drug-addicted inmates all the time at CJC. We have protocols for withdrawing from all manner of substances. With the exception of pregnant drug-addicted patients where we usually have to continue their narcotics to protect the unborn baby, we get all our inmates off their drugs.

I had one young offender, Alan Gregg, who received suboxone as part of addiction treatment on the outside. It wasn't being particularly effective, as he had relapsed several times. I started Alan on our detox protocol. Presley went ballistic.

This was terrible medicine, she asserted. Why wasn't this poor lad getting his suboxone?

"It's illegal," I replied. "You need special training to use it. I don't have it. The nurses don't have it. The staff that works in the rest of the facility doesn't have it. We can't use it. End of story."

"Well, by God, you *will* give him the suboxone!"

I didn't know what to say. "Undersheriff Presley," I explained, "the FDA says I can't use it. We have a detox protocol that we've used hundreds of times for just this kind of patient. He's not being neglected. This is my call, not yours. I'm a doctor; you're a cop."

"You *will* give him that medication!" she shrilled, her eyes taking on an unnerving reddish hue.

"I won't," I said. "I'm not risking my license just because you think you can ignore federal law. Why is it so important that this one patient out of hundreds that are in the same situation gets this special treatment from you?"

She wouldn't answer that question, but proceeded apace. "I'll get Dr. Eloise to prescribe it," she threatened, naming my predecessor at CJC, who now worked at a detox clinic that treated young Alan.

"I'm all atremble. Dr. Eloise has no authority to prescribe anything at CJC. She has no credentials here. You may recall that you fired her."

Presley sputtered and raged. She did everything but snap her broom in half. "You haven't heard the last of this!" And your little dog too.

She was right about that. Next day I huddled in Wendy's office on a conference call with Presley and the CJC lawyer, Mr. Black. Carl, our resident corporate sycophant, pulled up a chair.

The lawyer led off. "Dr. Wright," came the tinny voice from the speaker, "I understand you're not willing to give suboxone to Mr. Gregg."

"I'm not willing because it's illegal, Mr. Black."

"Would you be willing to talk with Dr. Eloise about this. She's an expert in the field."

"Expert or not, it's still illegal. There's no point in my talking to her or anyone else about it."

"What if it wasn't illegal," he oiled. I hate to pigeonhole lawyers, but this kind of I-know-a-loophole attitude just reinforces the weasel stereotype.

"If it wasn't illegal, we wouldn't be having this conversation."

He sprung the trap. "Have you ever heard of the three-day rule?"

We all looked blankly at each other. Even Carl. I guess I should say that Carl's face looked even more blank than usual. I wondered if the three-day rule was like the five-second rule if you accidentally drop something on the floor that you want to eat.

"No, I've never heard of the three-day rule."

"The FDA allows an exception in an emergency for a doctor without special training to continue a prescription for suboxone for up to three days."

"No doubt you have a copy of the exception handy."

"I do. I'll send it over." He did. I read through all the dire warnings about using suboxone including the section about the three-day rule. Buried as deeply as it was in techno-legal verbiage, I'm surprised anyone knew about it.

"Okay, Mr. Black. As long as you can declare this an emergency, I can continue the suboxone for three days. I'm assuming you can document this as an emergency?"

Black was caught off guard for a moment. "Well, of course it is."

"Not from where I'm sitting. Send me a signed document from your legal department stating that this constitutes a legal emergency, and then we can proceed."

"Oh, I don't think that's necessary."

"It is. Call me when you have it." When the FDA hit the fan, I wanted someone else's butt on the scaffold.

Eventually their legal department ground out a carefully-worded document saying they were pretty-much-almost sure this was an emergency. Of course by then Alan was halfway through detox anyway. No matter. He got his suboxone for three days and bonded out of jail, presumably to continue his narcotic odyssey with Dr. Eloise.

I thought that maybe at last we were done with who was the dog and who was the tail in medical. Not happening. I was summoned to Presley's office in the vaunted administration wing.

Presley was famous for her incoherent rages, and now I got to experience one. The tirade ended some twenty minutes later through sheer exhaustion with the proclamation that we could all work together harmoniously in the future. The hope was apparently based on Presley's assumption that I would toe the line, and let her run the medical clinic in the future. I doubt that I said a dozen words during the entire excoriation.

The reasons behind all this animosity were never clear, but it seemed to boil down to her desire to be in control of everything, plus a dose of personal vindictiveness against people in medical she thought didn't like her. Well, that was a pretty big club, and I never found out who she thought had done her wrong. It really didn't matter, as she was out to punish everybody in the line of fire. Speaking of which...

Twenty-eight

Abuse of Power

The sheriff is an elected post, and it's no secret that the sheriff, Terry Maketa, is politically ambitious. Since he'll be exiting the office in January 2015 due to term limits, there's noise that he wants to be Governor Maketa.

What did this have to do with the medical clinic? All the personnel at CJC were subject to witch-hunt paranoia concerning who was in Terry's camp and who wasn't. Undersheriff Presley led the inquisition.

I'm not a political person. I just wanted to come to work, do my job and go home, but the castle intrigues kept coming. I'd never worked in an environment so rife with threats and intimidation from the top. It seemed that every time I mentioned Maketa or Presley to one of the commanders, he'd quickly look over his shoulder and clam up. Everyone was afraid of losing their job if they expressed a hint of disloyalty to either one.

I couldn't avoid the drama of the sheriff's lame duck tenure. Newspapers contained a continuing blowup over Maketa's very public "investigation" of a political rival.

The subject of the investigation was a candidate for El Paso County Sheriff who promised a forensic accounting investigation of the department if he was elected. That could be embarrassing, as Maketa was reportedly sleeping with the comptroller that he handpicked to manage the $60 million department budget.

Maketa unilaterally rewrote sheriff department policies so they didn't apply to him anymore. Some key points included dating personnel he supervised and financial accountability for spending the department's money.

Since he'd been spouting off about the investigation of his political rival, the *Colorado Springs Gazette* asked Maketa about not adhering to the department's policy that forbids discussing Internal Affairs investigations. Maketa said, "You know who I am? The sheriff. You know who wrote those policies? Me. I can do with them whatever I want." Well, excuse me.

Following this, hubris uncontained, he took on his own deputies. Annually for the past twenty years the sheriff's office nominates a street-level cop for the One Hundred Club, a prestigious recognition for first responders who go above and beyond the call of duty.

This year Maketa nominated himself.

Well, not exactly. He had Presley do it. Since she couldn't drum up any support for her ambition to take Maketa's place, maybe she was looking to be Lieutenant Governor.

When the command staff met to present their nominees from the ranks of deputies they felt qualified, Maketa left the room. Before anyone could present their picks, Presley said it was time to vote, and they should pick the sheriff.

Despite the ensuing awkward silence, none had the courage to tell Presley and the sheriff to take a hike. Finally one of the commanders said, "Why are we even bothering to take a vote? No one is going to vote against him." Maketa's nomination was unanimous.

The winner gets a gold watch presented at a fundraiser for the families of fallen first responders. The *Gazette* got wind of the hijacking. "I think it's crap," said one of the pressured division commanders, who remained anonymous for fear of losing his job. "This is an award that is supposed to be for line-level guys, not someone behind a desk."

Apparently not satisfied with giving himself the award, Maketa announced his intention to fire two commanders who demonstrated "lack of character" in commenting to the newspaper about sheriff's office business. Of course, that was what Maketa had been doing for months.

Good to his word, Maketa had not two but three of his command staff walked out of CJC. These are some of the top guys in the department, summarily and publicly fired for political reasons. Someone here certainly demonstrated lack of character. Enjoy the gold watch, Terry.

If you've never witnessed being "walked out" of a facility, you can't really appreciate the humiliation. It's an ambush. The victim is working at his desk when two deputies come in. They tell him to not touch his computer or anything else. Then, in front of all his colleagues and co-workers, they confiscate his credentials and key card and parade him wordlessly like a felon to the door of CJC, where he's dumped into the parking lot like a sack of rubbish. Thanks for your years of service.

But wait. There's more. Amid a howl of public and private protest, Maketa announced that he was declining the award he gave to himself.

But wait again. There's even more. The *Gazette* followed up with an epic story detailing how Maketa had been boinking not one, not two, but at least three of his subordinates, including Presley, promoting all of them without qualifications to top jobs and top salaries. Then there were the joint trips to Breckenridge, Las Vegas, Florida, Reno, and Washington, D.C.

The story even included a nude selfie that Maketa sent to one of the women with the note, "Wish you were here." Geez, Terry. You'd think he'd learn *something* from all the stupid stunts pulled by the inmates.

Note to all potential felons reading this: Don't take a selfie when you're doing something illegal. Or immoral. Or you're likely to end up on the pages of the *Gazette.*

Now the FBI is investigating. I'm loving it. Ivana Trump said, "Gorgeous hair is the best revenge," but I'm thinking she missed the point here. Call me shallow, but there's something innately satisfying in seeing the haughty brought low, especially if they've given you a hard time during their reign.

The whole backstabbing atmosphere at CJC got to me a lot more than the job of running the medical clinic. I could fight disease, but not the gelatinous ooze of personal and political duplicity. Obviously I'm not ambitious enough. I suppose if I was afraid of losing my job I'd feel differently, but I'd rather lose my job than my self-respect. As a matter of fact…

TWENTY-NINE

THE BITTER END

"Doctor Wright, can you come back to the facility?" Carl, our resident corporate toady, sounded anxious, but cell phone reception in the hospital was sketchy.

I looked at the shadows lengthening across the park outside the critical care unit of Memorial Hospital. Friday evening visitors streamed into the front entrance. "Right now?" I asked. "Can't this wait until Monday?"

"This can't wait," he insisted. "How soon can you be here?"

"Look, Carl, my mother-in-law has had a stroke, and I'm up here in CCU with the rest of the family. What's so important?"

"I can't talk about it over the phone. Please hurry." He clicked off.

Well, hell, I figured a meteor must have pulverized the jail or some equivalent catastrophe. I explained the call to my wife, Mollie.

"You'd better go," she said. "There's really nothing you can do here but wait."

Envisioning dozens of bleeding and dead inmates, I scurried back to CJC. No smoke. No flames. No ambulances. Plenty of cop cars, but there always were. I went through security and back to medical. Wendy sat in her office, sorting through a pile of papers.

"What's up?" I asked.

"Beats me. I got a message from Carl that I needed to come back right away."

Just then Carl appeared and crooked a finger at Wendy. "Can you come down the hall with me?"

We both started to follow, but Carl asked me to wait and the two of them left for parts unknown. I called Mollie to check on any news, but things were still in a holding pattern at the hospital. I asked her to call me with any change and went back to the nursing station to see if they knew what was going on. Nobody did.

I waited and waited. About thirty minutes later Carl came back and motioned me to follow him. We walked down the main corridor toward administration.

"How are things going, Dr. Wright?"

"Not so great, Carl. I've got to get back to the hospital. What's the big emergency? Where's Wendy?"

He didn't answer, but showed me through the doors to a room in the administration wing.

"So?"

Carl fidgeted and wouldn't meet my gaze. "We…that is CHC, the corporation, is placing you on indefinite suspension without pay."

"What!!"

"We want you to know how much we appreciate—"

"Wait a minute. Indefinite suspension without pay sounds a lot like being fired."

"Take it any way you want," he said, crossing his arms.

"What's the reason?"

"It's a Colorado law that we don't have to give you a reason."

"Common courtesy would dictate otherwise. This place was going down the tubes until Denise, Wendy and I turned it around a year ago. CHC was going to lose their contract. We saved your miserable asses."

Carl shrugged.

I was losing it. "You brought me back here from a family emergency after everyone had left for the weekend so you could fire me? Is that about it, you piece of shit?" I'll admit my vocabulary was degenerating, but then again, I'd never been fired before, especially not by a slug like Carl.

"I want a reason," I insisted. "Who authorized this?"

"I don't have to give you a reason," he repeated. "This is what the sheriff wanted."

Ah! The light dawned. So this had nothing to do with medical issues. I was being fired because I wasn't on Terry's team.

Carl held out a fat, greasy, stinking, gutless corporate hand. "You're barred from entering the facility. I'll need your pass card."

This is why they don't allow firearms in the workplace. I swear I would have killed the little worm if I'd had one. I did manage to salvage some dignity. I ripped off my pass card, threw it under a heavy bureau behind him, and stomped out. So there.

And that was the last time I saw the inside of CJC.

It hurts to get fired, especially fired without a reason. CHC seemed to take pride in the fact that they didn't need a reason. I checked, and it was true. Colorado, unique among the states, passed a law that said it was okay to fire anyone at any time without any reason.

Wendy dropped off the face of the earth. I heard via the rumor mill that she was offered some kind of deal if she just shut up about the whole thing. She was well connected and often said that she had a lot of skeletons on her hard drive. Something like that must have happened because my former good buddy wouldn't answer my calls or emails.

A quality person such as me doesn't stay on the market long. I'd been working part time at a private prison and my old employer, the Colorado Department of Corrections, seemed happy to have me back running the infirmary at Territorial Prison in Cañon City.

I wondered who CHC had waiting in the wings to take my place. The answer: nobody. All they had was poor Gloria, the nurse practitioner, who was tasked with taking care of the whole 1,500-bed facility. Dr. Herr, my old equivocating boss, got to commute to Colorado Springs from Denver to cover. Serves him right for not having the guts to stand up to Presley when she needed to be slapped down.

It's not easy to fill these kinds of vacancies. Doctors don't line up to take positions in correctional medicine. It was plain that CHC didn't have a Plan B for when I left, but just caved to the sheriff's whim. That left 1,500 inmates without proper care, but maybe Presley was planning to see them in her office.

After several months CHC finally did get a physician from California to move to Colorado and take my place as medical director at the jail. She lasted three months before going on vacation and not coming back.

As I'm writing this, they're back to nobody again. I'm delighted. I know it's petty and mean-spirited, but that's the way it is. And I hope the waterlogged wall in my former office falls in on Carl.

THIRTY

PHILOSOPHY: ENTER AT YOUR OWN RISK

"America is the land of the second chance—and when the gates of the prison open, the path ahead should lead to a better life."

—George W. Bush

"In my country we go to prison first and then become President."

—Nelson Mandela

After nine years at this game of correctional medicine, I've got some thoughts on jails, prisons and in particular our system in the U.S. We've got lots of agendas when it comes to putting people behind bars, and not all of them seem very productive.

The first thing to remember is that most people in jails and prisons get out. They're your neighbors again, working (or not) in your community around you, your spouse, and your children.

It's a sad fact that the majority of people released from U.S. jails and prisons commit further offenses and head back behind bars again to repeat the cycle. What's wrong with these guys? Didn't they learn their lesson the first time?

Well, they did. They just learned the wrong lesson.

When someone commits a crime against another person, there's a lot of emotion on both sides. What we want is for everything to be put back the way it was, like nothing ever happened. In this world, that's not going to happen.

As the next best thing, society wants punishment of some kind. Just like when we were children, if we did something wrong and were punished, we'd learn to not do that again.

It seems reasonable, but it makes a lot of assumptions.

It assumes we're in an environment where we have a model for better behavior and encouragement to follow that model. Jail isn't famous for being a nurturing and supportive environment. Mom and Dad aren't here, but Professor Butch and Professor Bubba are. Guess what the lesson today is. Breaking and Entering 102 or maybe Sexual Predation 203. Most inmates don't learn new skills in jail; they learn new hustles.

So what do we do with thieves, rapists, and murderers? We might take a look at the Swedish model.

At over 700 imprisoned per 100,000, the United States leads the world in incarcerating its citizens. That's like locking up the entire population of Houston, Texas, the fourth-largest city in the U.S. It's more than ten times the rate in Sweden. The incarceration rate, while climbing in the U.S., is falling in Sweden, down a whopping 6 percent last year. Are we missing something?

If you look at prisons in Scandinavia, like Skien maximum security prison in Sweden or the island prison of Bastoy in Norway, we see a very different physical setup from supermax prisons in the U.S.

In Colorado's maximum security prison, Colorado State Penitentiary (CSP), inmates are confined 23/7 to individual cells with steel bunk, desk, stool and toilet. A solid steel door with a tray slot for passing medication and food is the only contact a prisoner has with the outside. Exercise is also solitary in a spare room with a chin-up bar as the only furnishing.

In Sweden, their prison rooms look like a Motel 6 with TV, computers, bookshelves, rugs on the floor, curtains at the windows and separate areas for reading and recreation. The prisoners, with some exceptions, aren't isolated, but are part of a community where each has a job with responsibilities and free time. They live in small, brightly painted wooden bungalows that accommodate up to six people.

Every man has his own room, and they share kitchen and other facilities. The idea is to get them used to the social situation they'll encounter when they're released. They earn about $10 per day and get a food allowance of about $120 per month. They fix their own breakfasts and dinners from items available in the prison's supermarket.

For these prisoners, loss of freedom is their only punishment. Administration puts emphasis on cultivating individual responsibility and functioning in a community environment. Recidivism is about 30 percent in Sweden and only 16 percent for those released from Norway's Bastoy prison, versus 65-70 percent in the U.S.

Bastoy's governor, Arne Nilsen, a clinical psychologist by profession, makes a point: "In the law, being sent to prison has nothing to do with putting you in a terrible prison to make you suffer. The punishment is that you lose your freedom. If we treat people like animals when they are in prison, they are likely to behave like animals when released."

Granted when I went to work at CJC I'd already had years of experience in corrections, but many start the job with zero corrections knowledge. In contrast, Norway requires three years of training to become a prison guard.

So is treating prisoners like human beings rather than people who should be shunned the secret to the Scandinavian success? That's certainly part of it.

A second feature is placing greater emphasis on reaching young people at risk for trouble before they get into the formal justice system. It's a compelling fact that 80 percent of death row inmates in the U.S. are products of the juvenile justice system.

Maybe these men could have been rehabilitated if reached early enough in their lives or if they were taught a different way when they started down the slippery slope of antisocial behavior. I don't know if this is true, but it's something we should think about in view of the Swedish model's superior results.

Although it's expensive to spend on preventive measures like education and social work to intervene in bad situations, it's more expensive to let the problems develop. One estimate claims that $1 spent in prevention saves $17 in later costs of property loss and incarceration, let alone personal misery. Like the old oil filter commercial said, you can pay me now, or you can pay me later.

Regardless of one's outlook on punishment, I think we can all agree that the best outcome of any crime is if it never happens. I'm way out of my depth proposing sweeping social change, but I think we need to rethink our concept of imprisonment. Is vengeance better than rehabilitation?

Any crime is horrible for the victim. The desire to lock up the perpetrator and throw away the key is strong. Society has a different stake. Most of the offenders are going to be out again, and we have an interest to prevent additional offenses.

Is loss of freedom enough of a punishment? Having worked around that atmosphere for nine years, I can vouch that loss of freedom is a major deal. If we could make the time in jail or prison actually productive for the offender, maybe it will be productive for us as well. Maybe treating criminals like human beings is an idea whose time has come.

Are the people in prison bad people? Sure, they've done bad things, but what about their status as humans? Now I'm diving into the deep end, and I'm not sure there's any water in the pool. What is the nature of evil?

If you peruse Amazon you'll find scads of books written on this very subject. Executive summary: nobody knows, but it's probably a combination of nature and nurture.

The psychologist Philip Zimbardo gave a TED talk last year on this subject. His definition of evil is the exercise of power to intentionally harm another. Works for me.

Ranging from the jail to the supermax prison, I've had patients with all gradations of the trait. Some I felt were "born that way" with gruesome stories back to early childhood. Others were recent converts to the criminal world and seemed to cross over the line prodded by a particular situation.

In the case of murderers, the distinction didn't make much difference to their victims. It does make a difference when I look in the mirror and ask, "Could I do that?" I'm afraid the answer is yes.

If I could kill someone, does that make me an evil person? Are my patients evil because of what they've done? Maybe we're all potentially evil. But I believe the flip side is also true—we're all potentially heroic.

People make bad decisions. No surprise here. If an environment of poverty drives someone to steal, is that evil?

Given the right environment, we're all capable of monstrous acts. Abu Ghraib and the Nazi concentration camps are only a couple of obvious examples of environments that encouraged evil behavior. Were these places populated with inherently evil people, or did "normal" people exhibit evil behavior when immersed in those environments? If you're not familiar with "The Stanford Prison Experiment," it's worth your while to Google it.

Here's the executive summary of the experiment: A mock jail was constructed in the basement of the psychology building by the psychologist, Philip Zimbardo. A group of normal Stanford students were divided into two groups, one prisoners and the other guards.

As the experiment progressed over several days, both groups unconsciously took on more characteristics of their roles, with prisoners becoming more defiant and rebellious and the guards becoming more draconian. Things started to get out of hand, and the experiment had to be stopped.

One conclusion of the experiment was that normal people placed in an abnormal situation will adapt to conform to their new environment.

Since the Inquisition, we've approached the phenomenon of evil behavior by punishing the individual. It isn't working all that well. I think approaching evil as more of a public health problem may be more productive. Fix the water supply, and not as many people get sick. Fix a toxic environment, and not as many people turn to crime as their best solution.

I think environment and the systems that create that environment are potent shaping forces. Does that excuse the murderer or rapist? Not a bit. But it can help us to understand how these tendencies develop and maybe grant us the wisdom to intervene earlier and prevent the later crime. An ounce of prevention. It might work. Ask Sven.

"Whenever you find yourself on the side of the majority, it is time to pause and reflect."

—*Mark Twain*

THIRTY-ONE

IT SEEMED LIKE A GOOD IDEA AT THE TIME

Most people are too polite to just come out and ask, but I can sense you aren't among them. The burning question is, "Why in the world would you want to give up a comfortable suburban medical practice to go work in a prison?"

I'll admit the answer isn't obvious. Like many physicians who do correctional medicine, I kind of drifted into it. First, a trip in the wayback machine to Indianapolis 2001.

Medicine is a prototypical burnout-prone profession. Doctors, especially surgeons, tend to be perfectionists and quite invested in achieving the goals they set. In 2001 I'd been in the private practice of neuro-otology for twenty-seven years. Neuro-otology is a hybrid specialty with a foot in ear surgery and another in neurology. I was good at it and enjoyed restoring hearing and relieving dizziness for patients who seemed appreciative. But…

As time went on I grew increasingly dissatisfied with the nuts and bolts of running a solo private practice. Reimbursement from insurers constantly depressed income, while increasing overhead squeezed the bottom line from the other direction. I worked harder but enjoyed it less and less. I loved medicine, but not the way I was practicing it. Long story short, I retired.

I've related in my other book, *Maximum Insecurity*, how I was offered a job at the Colorado maximum-security prison. When I first saw the ad, I dismissed it out of hand as something no self-respecting physician would ever do, but the idea just wouldn't go away.

I was looking for something different, and this certainly fit the description. Here was a chance to be a real doctor to people who likely needed one badly. Medicine could be interesting and fun again.

I took the job over the objections of my wife, Mollie. I struggled with not only the prison environment but also with learning general medicine all over again. The diseases hadn't changed, but treatments had, even though the

CDOC (Colorado Dept. of Corrections) wasn't exactly on the cutting edge of medical technology.

I thought I might do the prison job for a few months, just until something else turned up, but I got sucked in. I really was having fun again learning and relearning the practice of medicine. I found that the patients really did need me, although they would seldom say so. Despite dealing with a negative, abusive crowd, I began to develop the pride that flows from a job well done. My few months' commitment turned into nine years so far.

The experience at CJC was exciting and challenging, like running a third-world emergency room. The people I worked with in medical were great, striving to do their best in a difficult environment.

I can't be as charitable with the corrupt officers and weasel corporate types I dealt with. They are a stain on our society as much as the criminals I cared for.

I told Mollie I'd quit when it wasn't fun anymore. That's what I did with my private practice, and that's what I'll do with this job too. I've quit CDOC twice in those nine years because of interference from administrators and have now been fired once, but the job keeps pulling me back in one form or another.

So why do I keep doing this?

I got a note (printed here verbatim) from a prisoner, Eric Bartles, who was just being discharged from CJC:

Here is my info Please stay in touch. I don't have Anyone out here. Im a good person. This is my first time in jail it sucks. Please I can see you're a good person.

Keep in touch I Hope everything go's ok. Hope you have a good night.

Another patient, Robert Truaxe, was a fifty-something homeless man who drifted up to Colorado from New Mexico. Busted for vagrancy, he was a pitiful sight on his intake exam with matted hair and downcast eyes. In danger of permanent kidney damage from his diabetes, I spent a month's worth of appointments to get his sugars regulated, educate him about his disease, and establish a program he could follow on the outside. On his last appointment before his release he presented combed and clean-shaven.

"Doc, I just got to tell you if you hadn't gotten me fixed up, I'd probably be dead by now. I got me a place to go, and I think I'll make it thanks to you." He smiled and stuck out his hand.

About the Author

William Wright, M.D., currently Medical Director of the Cheyenne Mountain Re-entry Center, is a graduate of the University of Michigan Medical School. A private pilot, he is the holder of three black belts and instructor certifications in Tae Kwon Do and Aikido. He is a commercial artist (www.WilliamWrightArt.com) and plays guitar poorly in his spare time.

He lives in Colorado Springs with his wife, Mollie, and a variable number of fur-bearing companions. His first book, *Maximum Insecurity,* is a memoir of his eight years as the physician in Colorado's supermax prison. *Jailhouse Doc* is a memoir of his time as Medical Director of the El Paso Criminal Justice Center in Colorado Springs.

ACKNOWLEDGEMENTS

I have nothing but praise for the tireless and selfless work of the deputies of the El Paso County Sheriff's Department. They kept me safe in the medical clinic and still keep me safe in my bed at night. They perform a difficult and dangerous job with grace and humor. They tell good stories too.

They deserve a lot better recognition from the public they protect. They deserve a hell of a lot better from the command structure in the department, and hopefully soon they'll receive it. Good riddance.

My thanks to the nurses, aides and administrators in the medical clinic. There's a special place in heaven for those who dedicate themselves to serving the downtrodden and underprivileged, even if they are criminals, maybe especially so. Denise, Wendy, TMart, TPed, Stacy, Della, Janice, Sean, Carmelita, Mike and so many others who made my day lighter and my work possible.

I'm grateful for the prisoners as well. Willing or not, they gave me a chance to make a difference, and that is a magnificent gift for anyone, especially in the healing arts. Thanks and that will be three bucks.

To Mike Sirota, my editor for this book and my previous one, thanks are insufficient. Without his editorial talent and wise advice, these books would simply not exist. Hiring Mike is like hiring someone to beat you senseless in an alley, but when the bruises heal the result is worth it. Besides being a literary thug, he's also an extremely accomplished novelist. Treat yourself to some of his marvelous writing:

http://www.amazon.com/Mike-Sirota/e/B004HF9YSI

Finally to Mollie, who believed in me.

Thank You

Thanks for reading *Jailhouse Doc*. If you enjoyed it, I'd really appreciate you leaving a review on Amazon, Barnes & Noble, Kobo, iTunes or wherever you purchased the book.

An honest review from someone who has invested the time and effort to read a book is the best thanks an author can receive. If you liked this book, take a look at what it's like to be the doctor in a maximum-security prison in my book, *Maximum Insecurity*. It's on my website at WilliamWrightBooks.com or at online booksellers.

Thanks,
Bill Wright, M.D.